PRAISE FOR
LIFE BEYOND YOUR EATING DISORDER

"A truly inspirational read. Johanna's book is packed with sophisticated but practical advice on how to recover from an eating disorder. Most important, she offers hope to those who are struggling with these lethal illnesses."

—Craig Johnson, PhD
Director, Laureate Eating Disorders Program, Laureate Psychiatric Hospital
Past President, National Eating Disorders Association

"Johanna brings us an inspiring personal account of how her struggles with eating disorders impacted her life. In detailing the trials and tribulations she faced during her journey from illness to health, she forges an alliance with readers who suffer from eating disorders, offering them hope and helping them to become more amenable to seeking treatment."

—David B. Herzog, MD
Endowed Professor of Psychiatry in the Field of Eating Disorders, Harvard Medical School
Director, Harris Center for Education and Advocacy in Eating Disorders, Massachusetts General Hospital

"Johanna's warm, conversational tone invites the reader to join her as she openly shares her inner world, and the struggle and triumph of her recovery process. Compassionate, humane and wise, her inspirational story should not be missed. *Life Beyond* is a must-read for anyone, anywhere, along the journey of recovery from an eating disorder!"

—Wendy Oliver-Pyatt, MD, FAED, CEDS
Executive Director, Oliver-Pyatt Centers

"Finally a refreshing new voice speaks out about full recovery from eating disorders! I am proud to be on the same team as Johanna Kandel. If your life has been touched by an eating disorder in any way, you must read *Life Beyond Your Eating Disorder.*"
—Jenni Schaefer
Author, Life Without Ed *and* Goodbye Ed, Hello Me

"Johanna Kandel provides eating disorder sufferers the inspiration to believe in a future beyond recovery. Her exquisite use of metaphors, such as learning to use 'all the crayons,' 'opening the middle drawer' and the importance of 'floaties,' are so vivid that readers instantly understand what actions to take to move them into new spaces. She has indeed choreographed a dance of hope for all who read her book."
—Susan Kleinman, MA, BC-DMT, NCC
Dance/Movement Therapist, The Renfrew Center of Florida
Past President, American Dance Therapy Association

"Whether you are struggling, in recovery, recovered or helping a family member or friend through this difficult time, this is an amazing resource for you. Johanna's story gives each of us hope that not only can we recover from these illnesses, but each of us can help someone who may be struggling to find their way back to health and happiness."
—Allison Kreiger Walsh
President and Founder, Helping Other People Eat (HOPE Inc.)

"Johanna has taken a brave step forward to reveal her journey through an eating disorder and recovery. Not only will her story shed light on this devastating disease, but her tireless work to make sure all people are aware of the effects of disordered eating is truly commendable. Being a recovered bulimic I know there is a light at the end of the tunnel and I salute Johanna for her tenacity to keep the switch on."
—Kathy Kaehler
Trainer
Author, Teenage Fitness
Ambassador, the Alliance for Eating Disorders Awareness

"This book is an excellent navigational tool for the journey toward recovery from eating disorders. With fierce enthusiasm, numerous insights and boundless encouragement, Johanna carries the recovery torch high, illuminating pathways so others can find a life beyond their eating disorder."
—Anita Johnston, PhD
Author, **Eating in the Light of the Moon**

Life Beyond
Your Eating Disorder

RECLAIM YOURSELF
REGAIN YOUR HEALTH
RECOVER FOR GOOD

JOHANNA S. KANDEL

Founder and Executive Director, The Alliance for Eating Disorders Awareness

Foreword by Adrienne Ressler, MA, LMSW,
National Training Director, The Renfrew Center Foundation

HARLEQUIN™

Life Beyond Your Eating Disorder

ISBN-13: 978-0-373-89226-6

ISBN-10: 0-373-89226-8

Library of Congress
Cataloging-in-Publication Data
Kandel, Johanna S.
Life beyond your eating disorder:
reclaim yourself, regain your health, recover for good
Johanna S. Kandel
p. cm.
Includes index.
ISBN 978-0373-8922-6 (pbk.)
1. Eating disorders—Popular works. I. Title
RC552.E18K36 2010
616.85'2600835—dc22
2010002219

www.eHarlequin.com

Printed in U.S.A.

For all the amazing women in Monday Night Support Group.

You are my biggest inspirations.

Quand on veut, on peut. (When you want it, you can do it.)

— ROSALIE BELILTY, MY GRANDMOTHER

(MY HEALTHY VOICE)

Contents

Foreword

JOHANNA KANDEL BEGINS THE PREFACE of this wonderful book with a disclaimer, saying what she is not—not a psychiatrist, therapist, nutritionist or doctor of any kind. She does say that she is a recovered individual who knows the physical and emotional journey of those who struggle with an eating disorder. But, oh, Johanna is so much more than that, as those of you reading this will certainly realize by the last chapter. She is a visionary, an activist, a healer, a teacher, an organizer, a warrior, a negotiator, a mediator, an author and an optimist. She is an inspiration to all whose lives she has touched, but never has she wanted to be a role model to be admired, copied or looked up to. This book provides many tales of recovery to help readers understand that there are many paths to healing, each as unique as the traveler herself. The message reinforced here is that there is no room for competition or perfection in recovery—no glory in being the fastest, the best, the thinnest or the most popular. Recovery is a process and the right process is the one that works best for you.

I have been involved in the field of eating disorders for almost thirty years, specifically in the area of body-image treatment and training. I met Johanna when she was nineteen years old and a volunteer working at the International Association of Eating Disorders Professionals (IAEDP) Conference. Just as Johanna has changed and grown since that time, so has the field of eating disorders itself. We now know more than we ever did before about the complexity of eating disorders: their connection to other psychiatric disorders, the gender-biased risk factors, the role of the brain, genetics and one's temperament as variables, the connection between body shame and the culture, and the importance and effectiveness of complementary treatment modalities such as art therapy, dance/movement therapy, spirituality and yoga. Research has given us more information and more tools. We need to always keep the belief alive that recovery is possible, that no recovery is "perfect" and no one should ever give up. It may be useful to know that the word *recover* comes from the Latin and means "to bring back to normal position or condition." Therefore, the person we discover during recovery is not someone new, but someone we have once been, a person whole and integrated. Recovery needs to be viewed as a continuous process that allows for the development of a greater sense of oneself, not a definite end of symptoms.

Years ago I came across the following passage in the book *On Death and Dying* by Elisabeth Kübler-Ross. I share it here because I associate it so closely with the struggle involved in freeing oneself from the grasp of the eating disorder:

> It is not the end of the physical body that should worry us. Rather, our concern must be to live while we're alive — to release our inner selves from the spiritual death that comes with living behind a façade designed to conform to external definitions of who and what we are.

Like a vampire who takes the very lifeblood from the innocents who fall under his spell, so, too, the eating disorder takes the very life spirit of those who relentlessly pursue the seductive belief that their true selves do not measure up to societal expectations and substitute a "perfect" self in order to be acceptable. Recovery involves a reclaiming of one's true self, giving up the eating disorder identity, making peace with one's body, shifting away from negative self-talk, relinquishing a victim mentality and staying optimistic despite setbacks and difficult times. As Dan Millman, author of *Way of the Peaceful*

Warrior, said, "You don't have to control your thoughts; you just have to stop letting them control you."

Life Beyond Your Eating Disorder is a true recovery guide for individuals at any stage of eating disorder treatment or recovery. It is also excellent for families and friends to better understand how to provide support while maintaining their own lives. The book provides a candid, comprehensive look at the ups and downs of recovery and offers tips, resources, hands-on tools and strategies for breaking free from the distortions and beliefs that make up the world of the eating-disordered individual. The book is exceptional, as is its author.

Adrienne Ressler, MA, LMSW
National Training Director for the Renfrew Center Foundation
President, International Association of Eating Disorders Professionals (IAEDP)

Preface

MY MISSION

I learned this, at least, by my experiment; that if one advances

confidently in the direction of his dreams, and endeavors

to live the life which he has imagined, he will meet with a

success unexpected in common hours.

— WALDEN, HENRY DAVID THOREAU

I'M NOT A PSYCHIATRIST; I'm not a psychologist or a therapist or a nutritionist or a doctor of any kind. But I have been an anorexic, an exercise bulimic and a binge eater, and if either you or someone you love is struggling with an eating disorder, I can honestly say that I know what you're going through — maybe not the day-to-day details, but certainly the physical and emotional landscape of your struggle.

Perhaps one of the most important and startling things I learned both during my ten-year battle with an eating disorder and during my recovery is just how much ignorance, misinformation, fear and stigma are still attached to eating disorders even in the midst of the so-called information age. The entire time I was struggling and during my recovery process, I never knew anyone who had successfully recovered from an eating disorder. Truthfully, I didn't know if recovery was even possible. All I knew was that I was sick and tired of being sick and tired, so I decided to seek help.

As I began my own journey to recovery, I vowed to myself that if I were given a second chance at life, I would do everything in my power to dispel some of that darkness and bring eating disorders awareness and information into the light. I strongly believe that no one should have to struggle with or recover from an eating disorder alone.

No one should have to struggle with or recover from an eating disorder alone.

Eighteen years ago, when I first began to develop my eating disorder, I had no idea how many people had the same terrible disease. I honestly believed I was one of the very few. But here are the facts: according to the Eating Disorders Coalition, today, in the United States alone, approximately 10 million women and 1 million men are struggling with anorexia or bulimia, and 25 million people are battling binge eating disorder. Eating disorders do not discriminate; they affect men and women, young and old, and people of all economic levels. You need to know that anorexia nervosa has the highest mortality rate — estimated to be up to 20 percent — of any psychiatric illness. And only one in ten people with an eating disorder receives any kind of treatment. Those figures make me sad and are, quite simply, unacceptable.

As I began to recover and find my strength, I kept the promise I had made to myself all those years ago, and in late 2000 I founded the Alliance for Eating Disorders Awareness in my hometown of West Palm Beach, Florida. The

Alliance is a nonprofit organization whose mission is to prevent eating disorders and promote positive body image by advancing education and increasing awareness. To this end we do community outreach through talks at schools, we provide educational programs about eating disorders to therapists and other health-care professionals, we lead support groups for people in recovery and we do whatever we can to convince government officials that eating disorders ought to be a health-care priority. For specific information about the Alliance, see page 215. I believe we are fulfilling that mission with each person we are able to reach and inform that he or she is not alone and that recovery is possible.

I know how difficult the recovery process can be, but I want you to know that it is possible to get better—and it's definitely worth it! We all trip and fall along the way. But recovery is not about the trips and falls; it is about what happens after you pick yourself up. It's about getting back on your feet, dusting yourself off and moving forward, because that is how we learn. Realistically, neither life nor recovery is ever going to be a fairy tale, but we do have the power to create our own version of a real happily-ever-after.

---

*It is possible to get better—
and it's definitely worth it!*

Give yourself permission to imagine your life beyond your eating disorder. You will get to be present in every moment; you will get to feel; you will get to laugh. You deserve the freedom to live every aspect of your life.

Eating disorders can be very strong—mine spent years telling me all the things I couldn't, shouldn't or wasn't good enough to do. That negative voice isn't going to go away overnight, but there are many tools available to you as you recover to make that voice smaller and softer, and you need to gather and use every one you possibly can. This book is one of the tools you can use to free yourself from your eating disorder once and for all. As you read it, I hope the voice you hear in your head will be healthy, supportive and powerful enough to drown out whatever doubts you may still have about your ability to recover. I've gathered the tools that I offer here through many years of working with eating disorder practitioners, in support groups, walking next to people on their journeys to recovery and by becoming aware of what has helped others. And I hope that these tools will be as useful to you as they have been to me and to so many others. I'm sure some tools will be more useful to you than others, and that's okay. I wouldn't expect it to be any other way. The idea is simply to be willing to try, and if one thing doesn't work, try something else. Just don't stop trying.

---

*We have the power to create our own
version of happily-ever-after.*

As you read on, you will come upon the stories of many different people from many different walks of life who have recovered from eating disorders, and you will come to see that they have followed many different paths. And just as there is no right or wrong way to recover, there is no right or wrong way to use this book. You might read it from cover to cover, or you might choose to read a few chapters and ponder them for a while. You might even decide not to begin at the beginning but to pick a chapter that looks interesting and read that first. Whatever works for you is the right way.

Lao Tzu, the sixth-century BC Chinese philosopher and father of Taoism, said, "A journey of a thousand miles begins with a single step." Taking that first step toward recovery is really hard, and I admire you so much for taking this first step. You have come so far just by picking up this book. I know that together we can keep moving forward so that you, too, are able to create a new reality for yourself.

Chapter One

FOOD FIGHT

*Dedicate yourself to the good you deserve and desire
for yourself. Give yourself peace of mind. You deserve
to be happy. You deserve delight.*

— MARK VICTOR HANSEN,
AUTHOR OF *CHICKEN SOUP FOR THE SOUL*

MY STORY HAS BEEN TOLD MANY TIMES. The specifics of my particular journey may be different from yours or someone else's, but the basic story line remains the same. Since you've so graciously allowed me to walk beside you on your journey to recovery from your eating disorder, I think it only fair that I tell you something about my own experiences along that path. I don't expect that your experiences will be exactly the same as mine, but I'm sure that at least some of what I describe will be familiar to you. And, really, the point is that whether or not you follow precisely in my footsteps, you, too, can and will arrive at a place where your eating disorder is no longer the first thing you think about the moment you wake up in the morning, the last thing you think about before you go to sleep and what you think about almost every moment in between. My hope is that this book will help to make your journey a bit easier as you travel your own path.

Let's begin at the beginning. I was born and raised in West Palm Beach, Florida, but both my parents were raised in France. My father was a Holocaust survivor. When he was just four years old, his father was sent to Auschwitz. My father and his mother, my grandmother, were then separated from one another and went into hiding with different families in different places. Separated from both his parents for five years, my father missed out on much of the nurturing and early education he would otherwise have had during this critical time in his development. His father died in the concentration camp, but he and his mother were reunited after the war. Once he had completed his schooling, my father came to the United States to start a new life, returning to France once a year to visit his mother. It was on one of those visits that he met my mother, who had been born in Algeria and moved to France when she was eight years old. She was one of seven children in a family of a very poor and humble background; on many nights my maternal grandmother went to bed wondering whether she would be able to feed her children the next day.

---

*You will arrive at a place where your eating disorder
is no longer the thing you think about
the moment you wake up in the morning, before
you go to sleep and every moment in between.*

As a result of their own upbringings, both my parents were intent on giving me every opportunity to soar in every aspect of my life, but they also had very high expectations of me. While my mother was the nurturer, very affectionate and simply wanting me to excel at whatever I did, my dad was very much the perfectionist. He expected me to become a doctor, at the very least, or perhaps even a nuclear physicist. Because I was an only child, all their hopes, dreams and expectations were invested in me. Today I understand that if they pushed me, it was because of the potential they saw in me, but at the time their expectations translated in my mind to a belief that I just wasn't good enough to live up to the standards they—and my dad in particular—had set for me. But I tried. I always did as I was told, never gave them a hard time and put a lot of pressure on myself to do whatever I could to make them proud.

As a little girl I was extremely pigeon-toed, so my parents thought it would be a great idea to enroll me in ballet class to improve my grace and posture and help straighten out my feet. Much to their dismay, from the moment I got into that class, all I wanted was to become a ballerina. My mother continued to be supportive, but my father told me only recently that he had never expected me to become a dancer and had, in fact, been somewhat horrified by my announcement. Nevertheless, I started to dance at a local ballet academy and my training became very intense very quickly. By the time I was seven, I was already on a professional track. My parents had also enrolled me in various other classes, including gymnastics and piano, but my one true love remained ballet, and by the age of ten I was dancing four to five nights a week.

The summer before seventh grade, when I was twelve, I attended ballet camp in Chautauqua, New York, where I studied under a very well-known ballerina. I remember her saying that as dancers we needed to be "light as a feather" and the most beautiful ballerinas we could possibly be. Although she was undoubtedly talking about technique as much as weight, I immediately internalized the message that if I wanted to achieve my dream, I would have to be thin. If my dad had high expectations of me, mine for myself were even higher. Having internalized his message, it was no longer his voice but mine inside my head telling me that if I was going to do something—whatever it was—I needed to do it perfectly.

When I returned from camp at the end of the summer, I entered a new school for the performing and visual arts that had just been established. I had academic classes in the morning and dance classes in the afternoon. Then, when school was over, my mother picked me up and drove me and my friends to the dance academy of the local professional ballet company, where I was also taking classes. That fall the artistic director and the ballet mistress of the company came to our class and told us that they would be holding auditions and choosing a number of students to appear in that season's production of *The Nutcracker*. They said that they were giving us this heads-up because they hoped that we'd work on our technique and also lose a bit of weight before the auditions took place. I wanted to be chosen so badly that if they'd told me to go upstairs and jump off the roof to get the part, I would have done it. But beyond simply wanting the part, I was already, even then, the quintessential people pleaser. Because of my father's high expectations of me, as well as those I placed on myself, I simply didn't believe, however well I did, that I was good enough. As a consequence, I believed that if I did enough to please other people, they would like me, and I also believed that if other people liked me, I would find it easier to like myself. Therefore, my incentive to lose that weight was twofold: to get the part and also to please the ballet mistress and artistic director of the company.

If I wanted to achieve my dream, I would have to be thin. If I was going to do something — whatever it was — I needed to do it perfectly.

I was still small and prepubescent. I had no idea how to lose weight, but I was determined to do it. At that time, in 1990, fat-free was all the rage, so I decided that the thing to do would be to cut as much fat as possible out of my diet. I remember telling my mother that I was going on a healthy-food diet and would be eating fruits, vegetables and lean meats. (You know, this is something I must have read somewhere—probably in one of those magazines that teach you five ways to lose weight without really trying. Certainly, as a twelve-year-old, it wasn't anything I had come up with all by myself!) My mother, of course, thought that would be great. What parent wouldn't be happy to hear that her child *wanted* to eat lots of fruits and vegetables? I bought a fat- and calorie-counter book and began to look up the content of absolutely everything I ate.

They hoped that we'd work on our technique and also lose a bit of weight before the auditions took place.

I don't actually know if I lost any weight on my "healthy" diet, but I auditioned, and out of the fifteen girls in my class I was the only one not chosen for a part. The people from the ballet company took me aside and told me that the reason I hadn't been cast was not that I wasn't good enough, but rather that I looked so young. I was, in fact, one of the smallest and youngest in my class, but despite what they said, I believed they really meant that I was too fat and they were just trying to be kind. At that point I made a pact with myself: no matter what it took, I was going to get a part the following year.

I became very strict and rigid with my diet. I started to exercise even more, and I did lose some weight. People noticed very quickly, and they were telling me how good I looked, which made me feel great. But it also convinced me that I must have been really big. If not, after all, why would they be making such a big deal over the weight I'd lost?

*Despite what they said, I believed they
really meant that I was too fat.*

Some time near the end of my seventh-grade year, our health teacher showed a made-for-television movie about a young gymnast who was battling an eating disorder. I think that most of my classmates watched the girl in that movie and thought, *What is she doing? That's terrible!* But I looked at it and thought, *Hey, I can do that for a while. I'll just get down to my goal weight and then I'll stop.* I still thought losing weight was all about control, and since I was losing weight, I felt as if I were in control. Once I'd started, I just couldn't stop. My eating disorder took control of *me.* In retrospect, the danger of those movies (and we've all seen them) is that they provide anyone who's predisposed to developing an eating disorder with step-by-step instructions for how to do it really well.

Have you ever had a really bad stomach flu and had people tell you afterward how great you look because you've lost a few pounds? You might want to say, "Are you nuts? I was sick as a dog." But you might also get the idea that if you stuck with a restrictive diet awhile longer, you'd look even better. That was more or less how it went for me. I cut back more and more on my food intake, and the response I got from other people was, "Wow, Johanna, I wish I had your willpower. You can just sit there with a piece of cake in front of you and not eat it." Meanwhile, I was dying on the inside. People seem to think that anyone with an eating disorder simply isn't hungry or is indifferent to food, but that's the furthest thing from the truth. I thought about food all the time. My life revolved around what I was or wasn't eating, how much I was exercising and all the negative thoughts that constantly played like an endless tape loop in my head: *I'm not good enough. I'm not smart enough. I'm not thin enough. Nobody's going to like me.* Every day I was able to fight off the hunger, I felt I'd won—even though the only person I was at war with was myself.

I was dying on the inside. My life revolved around what I was or wasn't eating, how much I was exercising and all the negative thoughts that played like an endless tape loop in my head.

By the time I entered ninth grade, however, I stopped getting positive feedback for losing weight. The remarks of my teachers and classmates began to change. People started to ask me if I was all right. And to tell me that I looked really tired. I was already exhibiting various symptoms of anorexia—the paleness, the circles under my eyes, the sunken cheeks, the tiredness. I was tired all the time, but I still had the mental strength to get up, go to school, dance eight hours every day and maintain straight As. I was truly running on empty, but for the first time in my life I felt that I was really good at something; my eating disorder was rewarding my perfectionism. Even though it was the furthest thing from the truth, I believed that I was in complete control. In addition, because so much of my limited energy was focused on my eating disorder, I didn't have any energy left to think about anything else. I was emotionally numb, and I liked that because I no longer had to worry about whether or not I was good enough for my parents, for the world or for me.

Every day I was able to fight off the hunger, I felt I'd won—even though the only person I was at war with was myself.

Tenth grade was probably the height of my anorexia. I'd re-auditioned for several parts in *The Nutcracker* and gotten every role I tried out for, but now even my ballet instructor was very worried and started to express her concern about my weight. I still remember the day she took me aside and told me I'd lost too much weight. I felt so anxious and so guilty that I went home and had my first binge episode. I just wanted that feeling of anxiety to go away, and bingeing allowed me to stuff down the uncertainty and apprehension, at least for the moment. But almost immediately after, I would again be overwhelmed with guilt. Still, the anorexia continued throughout my junior and senior years of high school. I even passed out a few times—luckily never while I was driving.

I believed that I was in complete control.

Everything came to a head one evening in my senior year, when I had flown to New York to audition for a ballet company. When I got back home, still wearing my ballet tights under my jeans, I went into the bathroom to change. I'd always been very careful not to let people see my body, because I was so ashamed and uncomfortable in my own skin. When I looked in the mirror what I saw, although I didn't realize it at the time, was a distorted image of myself. If you've ever looked in one of those fun-house mirrors that makes you look extremely distorted, you'll know what I saw when I looked at my reflection. The only difference is that when you're in the fun house, it's the mirror that's doing the distorting, but for me it was what my brain thought it saw. I wore layers of baggy clothes and always made sure to change in the bathroom with the door closed. On this particular evening, however, the door was apparently not completely shut, and just as I was taking off my dance clothes with my back to the door my mother happened to walk around the corner and glimpse for the first time in almost six years what I had been so careful to hide. When she saw me, she started to cry. She began shaking me and screaming, "What are you doing? You're killing yourself!"

---

*I no longer had to worry about whether or not
I was good enough for my parents,
for the world or for me.*

Whenever I tell my story, people want to know, "What about your parents? Didn't they notice anything?" I admit that I sometimes wondered that myself; however, by that time I was driving myself to ballet class, and if my mother ever did see me in performance, I was on a stage, wearing a tutu and tights, with makeup on and my hair in a ballet bun. In other words, I was no longer Johanna. And the truth is that many people did know what was going on. I know now that several of my teachers had noticed my weight loss and expressed their concern to one another. And my best friends admitted later that they had been very worried but had been afraid to confront me because they thought I'd be angry and that would be the end of our friendship. In fact, while everyone knew I had a problem, no one quite knew what to do about it.

I'd always been very careful not to let people see my body, because I was so ashamed and uncomfortable in my own skin.

In addition, I'd become extremely manipulative and careful about keeping my secret from my parents, because I knew they were the only ones who could force me into treatment—and the last thing I wanted to do was let go of the eating disorder. It was my best friend and yet my worst enemy; it was what I knew and what I could count on. It was safe and, although very dangerous, very comfortable. I knew what it was like to have an eating disorder; I didn't know what it was like to recover—and what is known always feels safer than what is unknown. If there was a message on our answering machine from a friend's parent, I erased it before they got home. If my guidance counselor asked what I'd eaten that day, I'd come up with a whole list I could rattle off so convincingly that I sometimes got angry with myself for eating things I actually hadn't eaten. The truth was that my parents didn't really have any reason to think there was anything wrong. My mother had come from a family where every bite of food was cherished, and she'd been very thin as a young woman, so the idea that I would purposely starve myself was a completely foreign notion to her. In addition, I was dancing six to eight hours a day, so it would stand to reason that I was thin, and whenever I ate with my parents I managed to manipulate my food and make it appear as if I were eating. For people who don't have an eating disorder, all this may be hard to imagine, but if you have or have had an eating disorder, I'm sure you know exactly what I'm talking about. Those of us with eating disorders become experts at keeping our secrets.

When my mother saw me, she started to cry. She began shaking me and screaming, "What are you doing? You're killing yourself!"

In any case, that evening in the bathroom, my mother couldn't help seeing what I'd been hiding, and all I could do was to keep reassuring her that everything was okay, I was in control and I knew what I was doing. Still, she insisted that I see a doctor, and she went with me. To my amazement, when I got on the scale he looked at my weight and said, "You're really thin, but you're okay." Then he looked at my mother and said, "Just give her some of your good French cooking." This was 1996. Anorexia and bulimia were no longer secrets. They were listed in the *Diagnostic and Statistical Manual of Mental Disorders*; people knew about the death of Karen Carpenter; Tracey Gold had gone public about her battle with an eating disorder; and the seminal movie about anorexia, *The Best Little Girl in the World*, had aired on network television more than ten years before. But then, as now, there were many health-care providers who hadn't been properly educated about how to diagnose or treat eating disorders. And, of course, when a parent hears from a doctor whom she trusts that her child is okay, her inclination is to be relieved and accept the diagnosis.

So I'd dodged that bullet, at least for the moment. But about a month later my mother noticed that I wasn't getting any better. I still looked exhausted, with dark circles under my eyes, and I was still losing weight. At that point my mother realized that the problem was more serious than my simply being a little thin. She took me to another doctor, who was educated enough about eating disorders to diagnose my anorexia. When I saw the word *anorexia* on my chart for the first time, I freaked out. I was terrified that my disorder would be taken away from me. And, most of all, that they would make me gain weight! Although on one level I didn't want to live with my eating disorder, on another level I was petrified of living without it. It was the only aspect of my life that I believed to be in my control, and there was no way I was willing to give that up.

If my guidance counselor asked what I'd eaten that day, I'd come up with a whole list I could rattle off so convincingly that I sometimes got angry with myself for eating things I actually hadn't eaten.

I was put through a battery of tests that showed I had very low blood pressure, a very low heart rate, reduced kidney function and full-blown osteoporosis. You'd think hearing all that would have scared me into recovery, but no, it didn't. Then the doctor asked when I'd had my last period, and I just cracked up. He asked me why I was laughing, and I responded, "Oh, N/A!" "N/A? What does that mean?" "It means 'not applicable.' I've never gotten a period." "And you're seventeen and a half?" "Yes, but it's okay. I'm a ballet dancer. We don't get those." "But you've *never* gotten your period? That's not good. That's contributing to your bone loss and a lot of other things, too." My body was being starved, and we all need to eat. We need fuel, and my body was getting that fuel wherever it could—internally, from my bones, from my body fat and from my muscles.

The doctor looked at my mother and said, "Just give her some of your good French cooking."

The doctor then told me that I'd probably have fertility issues in the future, and my response to that was "Good. I don't want to get fat, anyway." Sad as that may sound, I simply had no sense of the danger to my health. I couldn't see past the present moment. In that moment all I wanted to do was dance, and I knew that I needed to be thin to dance. Honestly, it was the only reason I was living at that time.

On one level I didn't want to live with my eating disorder; on another level I was petrified of living without it.

Even though the doctor knew enough to diagnose me, he still didn't know how to treat me. His approach was to give me hormones and steroids to bring on my period and stimulate my appetite. Basically, he was going to fix me with medication. I was still restricting my food intake, but because of all the medications I was taking, I gained weight. In a matter of three months I doubled my body weight! Please note, I'm purposely not giving you numbers here, because I would never want my number to become a goal weight for anyone else. If you're struggling with an eating disorder, I can guess that you focus on numbers—the number of calories, fat, carbohydrates and proteins in foods you eat; the number you see on the scale; and the number you believe would be perfect. I also need to say right now—because I know that if you're reading this, you're probably thinking, *That's it, no treatment for me! No one is going to make me gain that much weight!*—that it is *extremely unlikely* something like that would happen today.

The diet gave me back my sense of control. My anorexia and the exercise bulimia came back with a vengeance.

For me, however, the doctor was giving me all those medications at a time when I felt completely helpless. Up to that point I had always felt as if I were in control, but now, no matter what I did, the drugs were causing me to gain weight. I was incredibly anxious and depressed, and I felt as if everything I'd worked so hard to attain, including my ability to dance, was slipping through my fingers like grains of sand. I was starving, and I figured that since I couldn't control my weight anyway, I might as well just eat and use the food to numb all those negative feelings. That was when the bulimia started. I never used self-induced vomiting, but I would binge and then purge with laxatives and compulsively overexercise.

At that point, I was about to graduate high school, and this was the time when I should have been auditioning to join a ballet company, but by that point I was too big to be a ballet dancer. Instead, I determined to use the next year to get myself back in shape and back on track. I stayed home and continued to dance at the academy where I'd been studying. By then I was in the most advanced group, so my classmates and I were often invited to take company class and sometimes also given roles in their productions.

Now I didn't know who *I was. My* only *remaining sense of identity came from my eating disorder. I had, in essence,* become *my eating disorder.*

At the same time, without telling my primary care physician, I also went to see a doctor who was a metabolic specialist and who already knew my history. I remember her asking me what I wanted more than anything in life. I said it was to dance, and she told me that she'd help me make my dream come true. Her way of doing that was to put me on a totally insane plan that involved my taking about thirty supplements a day (to date I still don't know what was in them) and going on a refined Atkins-type diet. Although I knew it wasn't healthy and was the last thing that I should have been doing, it gave me back my sense of control, and, in fact, I did start to lose weight.

As I began to regain a (misguided) sense of confidence, I auditioned and was offered an apprenticeship with a ballet company in Orlando. By then I'd achieved what the metabolic doctor considered to be my goal weight, so she took me off most of the supplements I'd been taking. I was supposed to be maintaining my weight, but once I was on my own again, I began to restrict even the meal plan she'd given me and I stopped taking the medications that had been prescribed by my primary care physician. My anorexia and the exercise bulimia, which had never really gone away, came back with a vengeance, and I fell back into my disordered eating really hard and really quickly. About six weeks later my mother came up to Orlando to see me perform, and, of course, she noticed how much weight I had lost.

If I were given a second chance in this journey called life, I would help others battle eating disorders so they wouldn't travel down the same path I did.

By then I was nineteen years old and really, as the saying goes, sick and tired of being sick and tired. Both my parents and my doctors had speculated that if they took ballet out of the equation, my eating disorder might just go away, and I actually thought so, too. After all, I really believed that the whole thing had started because I wanted to lose weight in order to be a more beautiful dancer. And I even remembered that when I was in high school, I'd look at the kids who were music students and think, *Wow, if I were a musician instead of a dancer, I could eat anything I want.* I don't believe it anymore, but at the time the idea that my dancing had caused my eating disorder seemed pretty logical to me.

I resigned from the company and thought that my eating disorder would go away immediately. Boy, was I wrong. In truth, dancing was the only thing that had been keeping me alive. Aside from my eating disorder, it felt like my only identity. Now I didn't know *who* I was. My *only* remaining sense of identity came from my eating disorder. I had, in essence, *become* my eating disorder.

I was alone in Orlando with nothing to do, and I was floundering. I'd never intended to go to college, and I'd never considered what I might do with my life if I wasn't dancing. I started to binge more and more, because I thought that was the only way I had to relieve the pain I felt. If you've binged yourself, you know that it has nothing to do with enjoying the taste of the food you're eating. Actually, in the moment, you don't taste anything at all. It's all about stuffing down (or numbing) and running away from any kind of feeling or sensation. After I binged, I felt awful and guilty about what I had just done. When I was restricting, I felt good about myself because I felt that I was in control. When I binged, I felt an enormous loss of control.

I called my parents and, for the first time, admitted to them that I really needed and wanted help.

I remember waking up at two o'clock one morning and realizing that I had no sense of who or what I was. My parents had been urging me to go back to school, and I decided to enroll in a psychology course at the local community college, thinking that I might gain some insight into what was going on in my own mind. It was while I was taking that course that I made another decision: if I were given a second chance in this journey called life, I would help others battle eating disorders so they wouldn't travel down the same path I did. Since all I knew besides ballet was my eating disorder, I determined that I would become a therapist specializing in eating disorders. After sticking my toe into academic waters, I went back to college full-time, entering the University of Central Florida in January 1998 and, in true perfectionist style, starting to follow an absolutely ridiculous, stressful schedule. (I actually graduated college in two and a half years...which is definitely not a healthy thing to do.)

I really had nothing in my life to focus on except school, and being focused on school became another way to numb my feelings. So that was where I transferred my obsession, taking more than the required number of classes. Given that I was in a cycle of restricting during the day and then, when classes were over, going back to my apartment and bingeing, my career choice was at the time somewhat ironic and, in retrospect, unrealistic. By that point I was wearing plus-size clothing, and to say that I was not a healthy girl (mind, body and spirit) would be the understatement of the century. But I knew that if and when I got better, this was what I wanted to do with my life.

In pursuit of my newfound career objective, I called a few local practitioners who specialized in eating disorders and asked whether I could become an intern or shadow them in their practice. They all told me that because of confidentiality issues, they couldn't allow me to do that, but one of them also told me about the International Association of Eating Disorders Professionals (IAEDP), an eating disorders organization that had just relocated to Orlando and was looking for volunteers. I called the executive director, Dr. Marie Shafe, who asked me to come in for an interview. She turned out to be one of the most amazing and inspiring people I've ever met in my life, and she urged me to volunteer. Before long, I progressed from volunteering to a paid position. I started to help out in the office, working on the newsletter and working alongside the director as her assistant. By that time it was the year 2000. I was in college, applying to graduate schools and working when I realized I was actually falling apart at the seams. I was realistic enough to know, after taking so many psychology courses, that I couldn't go to graduate school and learn to help other people until I'd helped myself. I called my parents, told them that I was putting graduate school on hold and, for the first time, admitted to them that I really needed and wanted help. I'd also confided in Dr. Shafe, and she helped me get into an outpatient treatment program.

Over the years I'd been to see many different therapists on several occasions, but until then I'd always told the therapist exactly what I knew he or she wanted to hear, and that was it. I simply wasn't ready to hear what the therapist had to say to me. I wasn't ready and willing to see a life without my eating disorder. I'd go to a nutritionist, take the meal plan I was given and throw it in the nearest trash can before I even got home. In other words, I manipulated everyone and sabotaged myself in order to maintain my eating disorder, which felt safe to me. The thought of giving up the eating disorder and going into an unknown place was much more frightening than maintaining the familiar, miserable as it was, and suffering the consequences.

I was still thinking in black-and-white, all or nothing. I was going to do recovery the same way I'd approached anorexia, wholly and completely. I slipped, as we all do, and boy, did I ever beat myself up.

But this was different. Now I had a nutritionist, a therapist and an entire treatment team, and I was truly ready to take back my life and get better. For the first time in my life I began to understand the feelings that underlay my eating disorder: why I hated myself so much, why I felt so undeserving, why I felt that everything had to be perfect. At first it was very scary to feel again after avoiding those feelings for so long. I didn't like it one bit, but once I began to understand that I didn't need to be perfect, that recovery wasn't going to be perfect, I started to breathe again. It wasn't easy, and I could not have done it if I hadn't already come to the realization that I *wanted* to get better and was ready to do whatever was necessary for me to get healthy. Up to that point, I honestly hadn't been willing; I just didn't want to. No one—including me—could love me enough for me to be encouraged to get better. I'd devoted ten years of my life to my eating disorder, and now, for the first time, I wanted to live, laugh and feel good about myself again. I even wanted to go on a date. At the time, I hated my body so much that I was literally avoiding any kind of contact at all with the opposite sex. Instead of checking out the guys, I spent my time sizing up other women and comparing them to myself—and, not surprising, I was always the one who came up short. I felt as if someone had taken away my soul, and now I wanted it back.

Never once in my entire life had I awakened in the morning, looked out the window in sunny West Palm Beach and said, "Today I'm going to become an anorexic."

I started to get better, but things didn't immediately become all better. In fact, my recovery process was far from easy, predictable or perfect. That was yet another hugely important realization for me. Initially, I was still thinking in black-and-white, all or nothing. I was going to do recovery the same way I'd approached anorexia, wholly and completely. I'd decided to get better and, therefore, I would be completely better immediately. I would be the Queen of Recovery—at least that was what I thought. Of course, it didn't happen that way; it simply isn't possible. I slipped, as we all do, and binged—and boy, did I ever beat myself up afterward. As was typical for me, I used my slipup as an excuse to keep telling myself that obviously I wasn't good enough to do even recovery correctly.

Slowly, however, my journey to recovery was progressing and I was gradually getting healthier, which meant that I was also seeing things more clearly—at least some of the time. Part of that clarity involved coming to the realization that I wasn't going to be able to counsel people with eating disorders in a one-on-one therapeutic environment while I was still recovering myself. That relationship would simply be too intense and triggering for me, and I didn't think I'd be able to maintain the proper therapeutic distance. In my heart, I knew I wanted to speak publicly about eating disorders because, as I was struggling with my own recovery, I really didn't have anywhere or anyone to go to for support. It was completely up to me to hold myself accountable and go to my treatment sessions. I had a wonderful family and wonderful friends, but none of them really knew how to provide the support I so desperately needed. How could they have known? I was living by myself in Orlando, I didn't confide in them, and therefore they had no idea what I was really going through.

There were several times when I could have easily lost my battle with my eating disorder, but I hadn't.

I didn't want anyone else to have to walk that path alone. I didn't want them to think that they couldn't get better. I wanted to walk beside them when they were going through the same thing I had so that they would know they were not alone. During the entire time I was in treatment, I had never known a single person who got better. I was white-knuckling it the entire way, and I wanted to make it different for others. I loved the work I was doing at IAEDP, but I wanted to get out there and bring education and awareness to boys and girls who were the "me" I'd been in seventh grade. I wanted to tell them that I knew what they were thinking—that they thought they were in control, that they could just lose some weight and then stop. I'd walked through that door, so I knew that once it slammed shut behind them, they'd have no way to get out. Never once in my entire life had I awakened in the morning, looked out the window in sunny West Palm Beach and said, "Today I'm going to become an anorexic." I wanted them to know that, and I wanted them to understand that if they walked through the same door I had, it might be the same for them.

During that first year of recovering, I remember talking to a friend on the telephone and laughing out loud. My friend started to cry and told me that she couldn't remember the last time she'd actually heard me laugh.

Once I'd made the decision to focus on helping other people through education and advocacy, there was another phone call to my parents. I told them I'd decided not to go to graduate school, after all. Instead I was going to start my own nonprofit organization. I was starting to feel healthy; I knew I could do it, and I wanted to give back because I'd been given a second chance. There were several times when I could have easily lost my battle with my eating disorder, but I hadn't. Now I couldn't take my recovery for granted; I wanted to share what I'd seen and what I'd learned. I realize now that my parents had been assuming that as soon as I got better, I'd be going back to school. Needless to say, they were a bit shocked. My mother was supportive, but my father was very apprehensive. He really wanted me to follow the traditional educational route, the one he had always wanted and planned for me. In the end, however, they agreed to support me for a year—which at the age of twenty-one seemed like a lifetime to me.

I filed the incorporation papers for a nonprofit organization in October 2000, moved back home in December 2000 and in January 2001 opened the Alliance for Eating Disorders Awareness. I called all my friends, my family, all the people I knew from treatment and various therapists, and I asked them all to tell me: If they were the parent of a child with an eating disorder, or if they had a client with an eating disorder who needed support, what kind of organization and what kind of information would they want to have available to them?

Based on the information I received from friends, family and therapists, I decided that education was the place to start. I believed that sharing my story and promoting positive self-esteem were the way to go. To do that, I would go into schools, start talking to kids and tell them what I had found out during my struggles with my eating disorder. My first presentation was at a local private school in April 2001, and I was terrified. In my excitement about starting the organization, I'd forgotten that I'd failed speech class in college because I was afraid to speak in public. Put me on a stage to dance before an audience of thousands and I was fine, but public speaking was something else. Nevertheless, I prepared my talk, got up before a sea of high school students and shared my story. In the end, it was the best feeling I'd ever had in my entire life. I'd found my path and I knew it.

---

*Now I can truly say I am recovered—
recovery is definitely possible.*

It's now been nine years of an unbelievable journey. I remember the first time, during that first year of recovering, when I was talking to a friend on the telephone and laughing out loud. My friend started to cry and told me that she couldn't remember the last time she'd actually heard me laugh. What an amazing day that was! I realized that, indeed, I could laugh again. And laughing feels really good!

If you've come this far with me, you've already gotten to the point where you are at least considering recovery. You've taken the first baby steps, and you're probably scared. As much as we all want to get better, it's frightening to give up something we know so well. When I was bingeing and restricting, I always knew exactly what to expect. I knew that if I did A, then B would happen. When I began my recovery, I had no idea what would happen, and for years I continued to tell people that I was recovering because I was still afraid to give up my eating disorder entirely. But now I can truly say I am recovered, and that recovery is definitely possible. Your path to health won't be perfect or simple or straight any more than anyone else's. In fact, it will be one of the hardest things you'll ever have to do. But I can provide you with the tools I've acquired over many years to help you persevere through the highs and lows of recovery. Some of my tools will also become yours; others may not work for you. And you'll probably be adding tools of your own. That's the beauty of the recovery process: it is unique to each individual. There is no right or wrong way to recover.

Your path to health won't be perfect or simple or straight. In fact, it will be one of the hardest things you'll ever have to do. But I can help you persevere through the highs and lows.

There will surely be slipups, but it won't always be so serious, either. We're even going to have some good laughs along the way. And the one thing I can assure you is that recovery is more than worth it—it is without a doubt the best thing I've ever done for myself!

Allison's Story

I first read Allison's story in the newspaper the morning after she won the title of Miss Florida. I was immediately struck by how eloquently she spoke about her battle with bulimia: trying to live up to unrealistic standards, living life after her recovery and her passion for using her voice to create awareness and change. She used the platform her Miss Florida title provided to educate others and bring attention to how serious and widespread the problem of eating disorders really is. When her reign was over, she continued her outreach by creating her own non-profit organization and traveling around the state speaking to students. I am deeply grateful that Allison has continued to use her voice throughout the years and that she now lives the life she imagined…eating-disorder free.

Ten years ago, my battle with bulimia was in full swing. My days were consumed by an illness I never expected or wanted in my life. When people think about eating disorders, they often think that they are a choice, but that simply isn't true. Eating disorders are not choices; they are mental illnesses, and they are also the leading cause of death among all mental diseases.

....

Eating disorders are not choices; they are mental illnesses.

....

In order for you to completely understand why my eating disorder began, I think it is important for you to understand a little bit about my past. I grew up in a very competitive home. My mom was a former national champion baton twirler, and by the time I was five, I was well on my way to pursuing the same goal. From the very beginning, I was a complete perfectionist and put a lot of pressure on myself. From pushing myself in the gym to expecting straight As on my report card, I didn't want to settle for anything less than the best.

One point I want to stress to you is that I didn't wake up one day and decide I wanted to be a bulimic. I vividly remember when my eating disorder started. I'd had a bad day at the gym and was really upset. For some reason I got so worked up that I actually threw up. It just happened; but in that moment something was triggered in my mind that eventually led to a life consumed by an eating disorder and some very serious side effects.

> I didn't wake up one day and decide
> I wanted to be a bulimic.

For three years my eating disorder was my secret, but by the time I was a junior in high school, I physically could not deal with it anymore. I went to my parents for help, but they didn't really know what to do. I became very angry with them for not being able to help me or give me what I needed, and at that point anorexia also came into the mix. By the time I started my senior year, my symptoms were very visible. I was extremely weak, I had lost half the hair on my head, I had broken blood vessels in my eyes, I had done damage to my esophagus from the bingeing and purging, I couldn't digest food properly even if I wanted to, and I was at a dangerously low weight. By November, I knew I couldn't live that way any longer. I went to my parents once again and at that point they took me to our family doctor, who diagnosed my eating disorder and told us that I would need to work with an outpatient treatment team. Together we found a psychologist, a psychiatrist and a nutritionist who would help me start to heal.

A major turning point in my recovery occurred when I left for the University of Florida the following fall. This was my opportunity to start my life over, but it also could have triggered my eating disorder again. I decided the best thing to do would be to surround myself with people who could help keep me strong and to get involved in groups that helped to prevent eating disorders. I volunteered at the student health-care center and started to tell my story. Interestingly, speaking out in public also helped me to help myself. I realized that by being open and honest about what I had been through, I was helping others who were either suffering or knew someone who was.

I realized that by being open and honest about what I had been through, I was helping others who were either suffering or knew someone who was.

At that point, I decided to start HOPE, Helping Other People Eat, which is now a 501(c)(3) nonprofit organization that works for the prevention and awareness of eating disorders.

I also wanted to give back to those organizations and groups that had helped me during my struggle. The National Eating Disorders Association provided a wealth of information not only for me but for my parents. Currently, my involvement with NEDA ranges from being a yearly NEDAwareness Week coordinator to serving as the inaugural chairwoman of the National Junior Board. I also lobby for insurance parity with the Eating Disorders Coalition on Capitol Hill and with the NEDA STAR Program in Florida, and I am an active supporter of the Alliance for Eating Disorders Awareness.

In 2006 I won the title of Miss Florida and went on to compete in the Miss America pageant. During my reign as Miss Florida, I traveled the state, educating all age groups about eating disorders. Over the last few years, I have spoken to more than forty thousand people about these illnesses and have made a commitment to continue speaking and reaching out for the rest of my life.

I truly believe that we go through things for a reason. Knowing how terrible it was for me to suffer from an eating disorder, I now live my life every day trying to prevent others from traveling down that path and helping those who are suffering to find the help they need.

Chapter Two

GIVE UP THE GUILT AND RECLAIM YOUR POWER

And the day came when the risk to remain tight in a bud

was more painful than the risk it took to blossom.

—ANAÏS NIN

IF YOU'RE ANYTHING LIKE ME—and the many, many people I've met giving presentations and in my support groups—you may have spent a lot of time beating yourself up and wondering how you could ever have allowed this to happen.

I honestly thought there was a perfect weight that would make me a perfect person.

In my case, there were fifteen young dancers in my class when we were told to lose weight. The others just lost a few pounds and then went on about their

lives, while for me the need to lose just continued and continued and continued. Each time I got close to my weight goal, I raised the bar and moved the
goal line back. I honestly thought there was a perfect weight that would make
me a perfect person. And each time I reached a lower weight, I really believed
that when I reached that next new lower number I'd be satisfied. I just chased
that rabbit—the illusive, perfect me—down the rabbit hole and found myself
in a totally strange world, one in which I actually didn't have any control even
though I had convinced myself that I was in complete control. And then,
when I tried to climb out, it was like walking through a hall of mirrors; I
couldn't find the exit no matter how hard I tried.

---

*I just chased that rabbit—the illusive,
perfect me—down the rabbit hole and found
myself in a totally strange world, one in which
I actually didn't have any control.*

Even when I was in recovery, I still kept thinking that I should have been
stronger, that I should never have let this happen. I should never have allowed
myself to slide down into that hole. Why, why, why did it happen to me?

Genetics—At Least Part of the Answer

One of the most exciting and enlightening moments of my life came when I
learned that research indicates there is a genetic component to eating disorders. Some people are born more vulnerable than others to developing an
eating disorder, and various researchers have linked the problem to the disrup-

tion of serotonin levels in the brain. Serotonin is a neurotransmitter, a brain chemical whose functions include the regulation of both mood and appetite. Some researchers have theorized that increased serotonin levels may leave people in a perpetual state of anxiety, leading them to gain some sense of control by restricting food intake. Low serotonin levels, on the other hand, could lead to bingeing on foods high in carbohydrates, which would temporarily raise serotonin levels and elevate mood.

In a strange way it was extremely liberating for me to read the following statement made by Dr. Thomas R. Insel, director of the National Institute of Mental Health, in an October 5, 2006, letter to the chief executive officer of the National Eating Disorders Association:

> Research tells us that anorexia nervosa is a brain disease with severe metabolic effects on the entire body. While the symptoms are behavioral, this illness has a biological core, with genetic components, changes in brain activity, and neural pathways currently under study.

While you might think it would be disturbing for me to learn that anorexia was a brain disease, it was actually validating to know that there was a biological explanation for my problem. And Dr. Insel didn't leave me feeling powerless, because he went on to say that "most women with anorexia recover, usually following intensive psychological and medical care." So, it is truly not your fault that you have an eating disorder. Even better, it *is* possible to recover—and you shouldn't be expected to cure it all on your own.

Simply telling someone with an eating disorder to "just get over it and sit down and eat" is never going to work. What are you supposed to say to that? "Oh yeah, you're right. For all those years I was struggling with anorexia the real problem was that I just forgot to eat, but now that you've reminded me I'll remember. Thanks!" No! Initially, I'd actually thought it *would* be that easy. I thought I could just sit down, eat a meal and not restrict, binge or act out. But, of course, it wasn't easy. It isn't, and it's not supposed to be. But now I have a valid, scientific explanation not only for why I'd developed an eating disorder but also for why recovery wasn't so easy.

It is truly not your fault that you have an eating disorder. It is possible to recover—and you shouldn't be expected to cure it all on your own.

Walter Kaye, MD, of the University of Pittsburgh Medical Center, working with an international group of doctors, has collected information from more than six hundred families in which two or more members had an eating disorder. In an article titled "Genetics Research: Why Is It Important to the Field of Eating Disorders?" Craig Johnson, PhD, director of the Eating Disorders Program at Laureate Psychiatric Clinic and Hospital in Tulsa, Oklahoma, states that these results may be nothing short of a breakthrough. They suggest that both anorexia and bulimia "are as heritable as other psychiatric illnesses such as schizophrenia, depression, anxiety and obsessive-compulsive disorders." And other clinical studies have also supported this evidence. One, conducted at the University of North Carolina at Chapel Hill, reviewed information from more than thirty-one thousand people in the Swedish Twin Registry and determined that genetics is responsible for 56 percent of a person's risk of developing an eating disorder—with environmental factors determining the rest.

As with almost all diseases and conditions, genetics may predispose us to being more susceptible, but our environment and lifestyle choices either increase or decrease our chances of actually getting the disease. According to Dr. Kaye, "We think genes load the gun by creating behavioral susceptibility, such as perfectionism or the drive for thinness. Environment then pulls the trigger" (*Journal of the American Medical Association*, Vol. 290, No. 11, Sept. 17, 2003). The problem, of course, is that if we know, for example, that we're predisposed to developing high blood pressure, we can avoid eating salty foods. But we can't remove ourselves from the world, and the world we live in is filled with messages and images that hold up thinness as a measure of perfection. All we can do is try to nurture our children's self-esteem and help them to develop a healthy body image.

As I thought about Dr. Kaye's words, I realized that when I started down my path to anorexia and bulimia, all I wanted to do was better myself, and I was in an environment that encouraged me to lose weight and be thin. I truly believed that if I lost weight I'd be a better dancer, and that was the most important thing in my life, the only thing I really cared about. So, not only my own perfectionism but also the environment in which I'd immersed myself were working together to put me at risk for developing an eating disorder.

When I ask members of my support groups whether there's anyone else in their family with an eating disorder, I see a lot of people shaking their heads no. And then I ask, "Well, what about your aunt Suzy or uncle Bob, who will only eat particular foods, has peculiar eating habits or is exercising all the time?" and all of a sudden their eyes light up and hands go into the air.

Looking back on it now, I can see that not only eating disorders but also alcoholism, depression and anxiety run in my family. I remember being a little girl and visiting an aunt, my father's sister, who worked for a large clothing store in Paris. She was petite and thin, and I recall her telling me that her secret to being skinny was to eat just one fast-food fish fillet sandwich a day. At the time, I didn't think, *Okay, I'm going to do that,* but it did reinforce the idea that weight was an issue and that thinness was something to work for. And now, of course, I know that my aunt must have had some kind of eating disorder — or disordered eating — herself.

In addition to what I observed in my father's family, my mother's sisters have also struggled with poor body image and have always been extremely conscious of everything they ate. So, in fact, there were eating and body image issues on both sides of my family. For me, the genetic gun was definitely loaded and just waiting for the environmental circumstances that would pull the trigger. I really didn't roll out of bed one morning and decide to be anorexic! And it's important for your recovery to understand that neither did you.

Make That Information Work for You

So, now you know you probably have a genetic predisposition that contributed to your developing an eating disorder. Does that mean you should just sit back and use it as an excuse to keep on destroying your health and your life? Absolutely not!

Eating disorders don't develop overnight, and getting better doesn't happen overnight, either. Everyone slips and falls. But eventually those trips and falls become less and less frequent, and recovery becomes a reality.

Giving up the guilt is entirely different from giving yourself an excuse. Now that you know your eating disorder has biological/psychological/social roots, you can use that information to release any lingering feelings of guilt you might have and direct your energy toward doing what it's going to take to recover. You just need to be aware that recovery isn't going to be simple, because the problem itself is complex. There is no one single factor that caused your eating disorder, and there won't be one single strategy that leads to recovery. I remember the mother of an amazing young woman in one of my groups saying that she simply couldn't understand why her daughter still wasn't getting better; she had taken her to see a psychiatrist, a psychologist, a nutritionist and a physician who specialized in treating eating disorders. To the mother's mind, since she was doing all the right things, her daughter should have been showing drastic improvement. I said to that worried mom what I say to everyone in my support groups: eating disorders don't develop overnight, and getting better doesn't happen overnight, either. Everyone slips and falls and gets up, then maybe even trips and falls again. But eventually those trips and falls become less and less frequent, and recovery then becomes a reality. It takes time, and it's a journey that doesn't follow a straight path.

Nobody's Perfect—Not Even You

Nobody makes the right decision every time. As an example, Anne Frank's *The Diary of a Young Girl* was rejected by fifteen publishers before Doubleday finally took it on and ultimately sold more than 30 million copies. *Chicken Soup for the Soul,* which has since spawned multiple spin-offs and become a worldwide brand, was initially rejected for publication at least 123 times.

Perfection isn't possible,
even for the best of the best.

And no one wins every game. In the 2009 season, Tiger Woods, arguably one of the greatest golfers ever, failed to make the cut in the Open Championship in Ayrshire, Scotland. At that point he could have said, "I quit. I've lost it. I'm not as good as I used to be and I don't deserve to be here." But he didn't, and two weeks later he won the Buick Open.

The great Michael Jordan had a lifetime field goal average of .497, which means that he missed more baskets than he made. Mickey Mantle had a lifetime batting average of .298, meaning that he had a base hit less than 30 percent of the times he was at bat.

The point is that perfection isn't possible, even for the best of the best.

To get comfortable with recovery, it is important to get used to the idea of living most of the time out of that middle drawer.

The illusion of perfectionism and having total control was probably at least partially responsible for getting you where you wound up in the first place, as it was for me. If you don't let go of that illusion, you'll just be setting yourself up for more of the same. I know, because I've been there time and again. At the first sign things aren't going as perfectly as you believe they should, you'll begin to think, *Okay, I'm not doing this recovery thing very well. I don't deserve it.* Or else you'll think, *Okay, I already messed up, so I'll just keep acting out for the rest of the day and start fresh tomorrow.* The positive strides you've made up to that point suddenly become null and void, and you almost start to believe that you deserve to punish yourself. You tell yourself, *I'm bad. I am not doing recovery well enough or the right way!* Not true! Just because you acted out at 9:27 a.m. doesn't mean that you have permission to act out again at 12:27 p.m. and 3:27 p.m.! You do not need to wait an entire day to continue taking care of yourself, because guess what? Nine twenty-eight in the morning is a new moment.

How Many Drawers Are in Your Dresser?

Several years ago, when I was having a problem making a difficult decision, a wise therapist suggested that I imagine I had a dresser with seven drawers. The top drawer represented the absolute best possible outcome (think fireworks)—perfection. The bottom drawer was the absolute worst. And the fourth drawer, midway between them, meant that things would be okay, manageable, relatively smooth sailing. Not every decision or action could possibly fall into the top drawer, but that didn't necessarily mean that it automatically fell into the bottom drawer—there was a drawer in the middle where things were *just fine*.

I loved that image and immediately began to think about how I could use it to help myself and others in recovery. In terms of the recovery process, the top drawer would mean quitting cold turkey, eating freely with no fears or reservations. You'd be healthy and happy, and all the little birdies would be singing. The bottom drawer would be: *This is too hard. I can't do it. It doesn't work. Failure. I give up!* Every negative thought you'd ever had about recovery would go in that bottom drawer. And the middle drawer would represent accepting the fact that the recovery process wouldn't be perfect or easy; you might trip and fall from time to time, but you'd be able to pick yourself up and keep moving forward.

Sometimes you will be working out of one drawer, while other times you will be working out of another. To get comfortable with recovery, it is important to get used to the idea of living most of the time out of that middle drawer. But what about those other four drawers, the ones we haven't talked about yet? They represent those gray areas, times when you do a bit better or worse than okay. And the drawers are there to remind you that you're not going to be thinking only in black-and-white anymore; there are other options.

Remember those drawers; they will reappear in future chapters.

In her book *Traveling Mercies* Anne Lamott writes, "I took a long, deep breath and wondered as usual, where to start. You start where you are, is the secret of life. You do the next right thing you can see. Then the next." Each moment presents a new opportunity to do the next right thing. Pick yourself up, dust yourself off and keep looking ahead, not back. You *can* do this! Believe in yourself and focus on your successes, not your failures; after all, you made it to 9:27 a.m., didn't you?

Just because you acted out at 9:27 a.m. doesn't mean that you have permission to act out again at 12:27 p.m. and 3:27 p.m.! Nine twenty-eight in the morning is a new moment. It is a new opportunity.

Realizing that you're not perfect is liberating. I know it was for me. Trying to be perfect is exhausting. Having an eating disorder is exhausting. Honestly, it is all exhausting. Aside from the fact that you're not nourishing your body or your brain, the constant obsessive thoughts and need to achieve, the black-and-white of it all, is totally exhausting, because it just never, never stops. So when you no longer have to be perfect, what freedom there is in continuing to move forward with your recovery! What energy you feel!

Realizing that you're not perfect is liberating.

Learn to Hit the Pause Button

One trick that helped me and that seems to help the people in my support groups is learning to "pause" their negative, obsessive thoughts. When those thoughts are threatening to overwhelm you, visualize yourself standing in front of a DVD or VCR player. (For those of you who are not familiar with VCRs, they're what we used to watch recordings on our televisions before we had DVD and Blu-ray players.) At first you will probably be a bit overwhelmed by the notion of completely ejecting your negative thoughts from your brain. So, rather than being scared to death to hit the Eject button, you can imagine yourself pressing the Pause button to give yourself a break from the constant negative thoughts playing on the tape in your head. After you've been doing that more and more often, you'll be able to hit the Stop button. Then, when you are ready, you'll get to the point where you can press the Eject/Erase button and get rid of those negative thoughts for good.

You may find that you've been doing a great job pausing those negative thoughts for a while and then a stressor you hadn't planned on arrives. When that happens, you may find that it's harder to pause the VCR for a while. But actually, that's okay, because it's only temporary. Take a few deep breaths, remind yourself how far you've come already and sooner rather than later you will get back to pausing again. In fact, once you've dealt with a few of those stressors (whatever they are), it will be easier to get back on track, because you'll know from experience that the stressful situation will pass. It's a process, and it works.

PS: Once you've ejected and erased a negative thought, get out your imaginary hammer and smash the cassette as many times as you need to in order to destroy that tape forever.

If you still think you should simply be able to quit cold turkey, you haven't yet given up thinking of yourself as having some kind of superpower. If you think that's the only way to do it, you'll sabotage yourself from the start. Imagine yourself standing at the base of a big, tall mountain and looking up. If someone told you to climb straight up to the top of that mountain without the aid of ropes, harnesses, grips or proper climbing shoes, how would you feel? Overwhelmed? Wouldn't you feel that you were being asked to do the impossible? If so, you'd be right. But if you were told you could get to the top by walking in a spiral around the mountain at a much less steep angle of ascent, that there would be maps, rest stops, guides and water stations along the way, that you might slip backward from time to time but there would always be someone to catch and support you, you'd probably feel a lot better about starting the climb. It might be a longer journey, but you'd know that the summit was ultimately within your reach and that you could get there.

Change Doesn't Come Easy

Making the decision to give up the guilt and reclaim your true power means that you'll be moving into unknown territory, and, honestly, that can be a bit scary. One of the many factors contributing to eating disorder development is the desire to escape all those overwhelming feelings and complicated emotions that come at us every day. If we feel inadequate or undeserving or anxious, bingeing might bury those feelings, and restricting can give us an illusory sense of control. We know that if we do A, then B will happen. If we've been doing that for years and now we start to do something different, it will be uncomfortable simply because it's new and we don't know exactly what's going to happen. That's why we need to take baby steps. We need to give ourselves time to get comfortable with the idea that we *can* do things differently. We can't change everything about ourselves all at once—but we do have the power to change, and we deserve to.

Lighten Your Load

As you begin your climb up Recovery Mountain, lightening your load will make it a lot easier.

Those of us with eating disorders share a tendency to take on too many burdens. It's as if we were going through life carrying a backpack full of really heavy bricks, and, trust me, that makes it awfully difficult to keep on moving forward. (Some people in recovery have even said that it can feel as if they're lugging an entire U-Haul truck behind them.) Some of the bricks—such as avoidance, fear of confrontation, self-loathing, people pleasing, perfectionism, to name a few—are of our own making. But they were not created in a day. Sometimes we buy into being what we think we are supposed to be (like a people pleaser). And sometimes, even though we may be aware that it's not in our best interest, we volunteer to carry other people's bricks without ever being asked. If someone else is having a bad day, do you tend to think it's your fault? If there is strife in your family, do you believe it's your job to keep the peace? Are you constantly trying to live up to someone else's expectations?

As you travel the path to recovery, make some time to take an inventory of what you're carrying in your backpack. Which of those bricks truly belong to you and which belong to someone else? Some of those we tend to take on for others are:

- **Our parents' relationship**
- **Maintaining peace in our family**
- **Being responsible for other people's actions, destructive behaviors and feelings**

When you're ready, start to chip away at those bricks one by one and return the ones that don't belong to you to their rightful owners, or just throw them away. Give yourself permission to walk away from the unnecessary burdens you have now unloaded. They are no longer your burdens to carry. As you do this, your own load will become a lot lighter and you'll make the ascent a lot easier, and you will also be making room to accept support and take on behaviors that empower and support your own health and wellness.

PS: Consider investing in a nice sturdy (imaginary) lock for your backpack so that, in the future, no more unwanted bricks can mysteriously find their way inside.

*We can't change everything about ourselves
all at once—but we do have the power
to change, and we deserve to.*

I often ask the people in my groups what it would mean to them to declare independence from their eating disorder. The answers I get are both extremely humbling and extremely empowering:

- To give up control and just be able to live
- To let go of the negative and make room to bring in the positive
- To be in the present and an active participant in my own life
- To be willing to just "be"
- To believe in myself
- To like myself
- And, yes, even to embrace change

As you take those steps toward independence, think about what being free of your eating disorder would mean to you. Write down your goals, keep them in your mind's eye and return to them often, particularly when the inevitable slipups occur and you feel as if you might slide right back down the mountain. Remember, even if you do slide backward a bit, you won't go back to where you started. You'll be somewhere farther along the trail to recovery. You'll already have had the experience of meeting some of your goals, so the road will be more familiar, less frightening and, hopefully, a bit easier to navigate.

Chapter Three

LEARN TO USE ALL THE CRAYONS
IN YOUR BOX

If you want the rainbow, you gotta put up with the rain.
— DOLLY PARTON

AFTER LIVING WITH THE REALITY of my eating disorder for so long, I initially thought that my recovery would follow the same trajectory—all or nothing, black or white. Each day would be either the best of days or the worst of days. I didn't even want to think about the fact that some days might be gray or just okay. Honestly, living with the okay was unacceptable. It just didn't feel good enough to me.

What the black-and-white thinking that characterizes an eating disorder teaches us is that if we do what we must to maintain our false sense of control, it's going to feel really good. It will be a "yay" day. And if we do something wrong, it will be horrible and scary. Fear—of the unknown, of not being capable, of feeling the pain and then letting it go away, or of just feeling anything at all—may be the biggest and scariest obstacle standing in the way of anyone's recovery.

*Fear—of the unknown, of not being capable,
of feeling the pain and then letting it go away,
or of just feeling anything at all—may be
the biggest and scariest obstacle standing
in the way of anyone's recovery.*

If we want to move forward with our recovery we need to acknowledge the fear, stop thinking in black-and-white and get comfortable with the idea that we won't always be comfortable. Some days we'll feel great, unfortunately other days we'll feel awful, but most days will be somewhere in between… some shade of gray. That's what those dresser drawers we talked about in the previous chapter are all about.

*Some days we'll feel great, unfortunately other
days we'll feel awful, but most days will be
somewhere in between…some shade of gray.*

How Many Crayons Are in Your Box?

Take a moment to think about your favorite painting. Now, can you imagine what it would look like if it were painted only in black and white? How would van Gogh's *The Starry Night* or *Sunflowers*, or Klimt's *The Kiss*, look in those two colors? Do you think they—or your own favorite painting—would still be hung in museums and decorating the walls of so many apartments and dorm rooms?

What Would You Do If You Weren't Afraid?

If a genie appeared and told you that for one day you would know no fear, what would you do? I have posed that question to members of my support group many times, and their answers are always both insightful and enlightening. No one says he or she is going to climb up the outside of the Empire State Building like Spider-Man or bungee jump off a bridge. Instead their answers are more like:

I'd take more risks.
I'd use my voice.
I'd take care of myself.
I would allow myself to dream.
I would nourish myself.

I would tell myself I was worth it.
I would do what I really wanted to do.
I would stand up for myself.
I would believe in myself.

What are you most afraid of, and what would you do if you had no fear for even one day?

Take a moment to write down all the things you would do if you weren't afraid. Make sure to keep your eating disorder and negative voice out of the list-making process. When you have completed your list, make sure to leave plenty of extra room below. You will need that room to add to the list as you accomplish some of your goals and start to create new ones. And know that one day down the road to recovery, doing those things won't seem as impossible as they might now. In fact, you will be able to look at your list and realize how far you've come. Remember, no one is expecting you to conquer all your fears yesterday. This is a journey that starts with your readiness to imagine your life without an eating disorder, and your willingness to try something new and different.

PS: As you make your way through your list, feel free to invest in a package of gold stars. Place a gold star next to each of your accomplishments. You deserve that reinforcement.

It's the variety and shades of color that make the world vibrant, exciting and beautiful. Even a black-and-white photograph isn't really black and white; it also has many different shades of gray. The smallest Crayola crayon box has 8 different colors; the biggest box has 120, and there are probably many more colors that Crayola hasn't even included in that box. The problem is that when we have an eating disorder, we don't see all those colors. In fact, we don't even conceive of their existence. The only crayons in our box are the black one and the white one. Not a very large or interesting box, is it?

When we have an eating disorder, we don't see all those colors. The only crayons in our box are the black one and the white one.

On the day I first committed to my recovery, I can honestly say that I had only two crayons in my box: one black and one white. I went to my nutritionist equipped with my white crayon. I was ready to start taking care of myself. I took the meal plan she gave me, went home and laid it out on the table. Then I stared at it for a while. I was really scared.

In fact, I panicked. But I knew I needed to do it. The perfectionist in me wanted to be a model client so that my nutritionist would be proud of me. For three days I tried to follow the plan to the letter. I nourished myself and took the risks the nutritionist wanted me to take—giving up some of my sacred safe foods and trying some that scared the living daylights out of me. I was frightened, anxious and extremely overwhelmed, but I did it. You know what's coming next, don't you? It just became too much, and I acted out. I slipped and immediately felt like a failure. My negative voice took over and I, the obedient student, listened.

I reverted to my unhealthy behaviors, and in my mind that slip immediately negated everything I'd accomplished in the previous three days. My white crayon was now nowhere to be found. The only color I had to work with was black.

I slipped and immediately felt like a failure. My white crayon was now nowhere to be found. The only color I had to work with was black.

For me, it had always been that way. I remember the first time I got a B on a test in college; I thought the world had come to an end. When I got my test paper back and looked at the grade, at first I couldn't comprehend what I saw. I recall showing the paper to my friend, who said, "Johanna, you got a B. That's great." And I said, "No, it's not. It's a B!" "But," she said, "you got forty-two out of fifty questions right." "No," I argued, "I got eight wrong!" It was a while before I could accept the fact that getting a B wasn't the end of the world and that I wasn't going to fail the course because I wasn't perfect.

It took a lot of faith, taking risks while white-knuckling my way through many more scary situations and many, many baby steps, but eventually I was able to accept the idea that life (and especially recovery)—mine, yours and everyone else's—isn't always black or white. More often than not, it's some other color in between.

Eventually I was able to accept the idea that life (and especially recovery) — mine, yours and everyone else's — isn't always black or white. More often than not, it's some other color in between.

As you embark on your own unique road to recovery, you probably won't be ready to use the boldest colors right away — and maybe you'll never be comfortable with those colors. But you may be able to get comfortable with using just the ecru or the dark brown crayon. And then, sometimes you're going to feel really great, and you'll want to be shocking pink or turquoise blue. Some days won't be so great, and on those days you'll feel sort of gray or sandy. Most days, however, you'll actually be comfortable using your beige crayon. (Believe it or not, beige goes very nicely with almost every other color.) Realistically, life is going to be okay about 90 percent of the time.

Ninety percent of the time you'll be living out of that middle drawer and probably won't feel like the brightest crayon in the box — and that's just fine. In fact, we sincerely need to learn to get comfortable and be okay with being okay, because okay really is good enough!

Maybe the idea of having to choose among 120 colors will be too overwhelming at first. If so, just start with an 8-pack of crayons and work yourself up from there. Even if you're never comfortable with all 120 colors in the biggest box, they will still be there for you to use if you should choose to do so. The key is to commit yourself to the process and know that even if you can't see it yet, you really do have access to all the colors in the crayon box of life. They key is making the choice to use your colors, perhaps trying them out one new color at a time.

PS: *These days I am proud to say that the colors in the box of my life now include Crayola's burnt sienna, mauvelous and purple heart. I wonder what colors will be in your box.*

Ninety percent of the time you'll be living out of that middle drawer and probably won't feel like the brightest crayon in the box—and that's just fine. We sincerely need to learn to get comfortable and be okay with being okay, because okay really is good enough!

Getting Comfortable Takes Practice

Letting go of your fear, beginning to think in color, means that you'll be embarking on something totally different, which can feel like standing on the edge of a pool filled with freezing cold water. You have three choices: you can walk away and avoid the pool altogether, you can cannonball right in, or you can immerse yourself gradually as you get used to the temperature of the water. Avoiding the pool completely means that you won't have to feel the freezing cold water, but neither will you be giving yourself the chance to see if you actually might enjoy the swim. If you cannonball into the pool, the sudden cold might be such a shock that you leap right out, never to return again. But if you slowly immerse yourself, you can start by dipping one foot, then two feet, then getting wet up to your knees and maybe sitting on the edge of the pool until you are ready to swim. All I ask is that you be willing to take a chance and dip your big toe into the pool of recovery so that you can start getting comfortable with the process. First things first, and then the process begins.

Add a Little Color to Your Life

Think about a time when you were confronted with a situation that made you feel uncomfortable. Perhaps you were supposed to go out to dinner with friends. All you could imagine was that you'd either think of some excuse to avoid the situation and, therefore, stay in control (the all-white choice) or you'd go, eat all the wrong foods and hate yourself afterward (the all-black choice).

Now consider how you might use some of the other crayons in your box. You might work out a plan of action with your treatment team to make sure you were comfortable. You might look at the menu online in advance and decide (maybe with the help of your nutritionist) what you were going to eat. Either option would introduce a bit of gray and shade your black-and-white view of the situation just a bit.

Imagine for a minute that you're right-handed and you break your right hand. You can either (a) decide that you're not going to write at all or (b) determine that you're going to learn to write with your left hand. At first that's going to feel really weird, and your writing probably will not be very legible. But the more you practice, the more comfortable it will feel and the more legible your writing will become. Remember that when you were a child first learning to write, your dominant hand didn't do so well, either! It probably felt a lot like what writing with the wrong hand would feel like now. But as you practice and grow accustomed to doing something different, over time it becomes second nature.

As you continue to put one foot in front of the other down the road of recovery, it might feel awkward at first, but the more you stick to your healthy path, the more comfortable it will become.

That's probably more or less the way you learned to be secure in your eating disorder. I know that initially acting out with food didn't make me feel great. In fact, I actually felt really bad. But then, after a while, it started to feel comfortable, safe, like second nature. I was rewarded with numbness but lost out on the feelings. And it's going to be the same with recovery. As you continue to put one foot in front of the other down the road of recovery, it might feel awkward at first, but the more you stick to your healthy path, the more comfortable it will become. You will be rewarded; you just need to give it a chance. You really do deserve to give yourself that chance.

You need to give yourself permission to be vulnerable because that's also giving yourself permission to succeed.

To give yourself a chance, you must initially give yourself permission to take a risk and perhaps fail—at least the first time. You need to give yourself permission to be vulnerable because, in fact, that's also giving yourself permission to succeed. If you're constantly protecting yourself from failure or from being hurt, you're truly cutting yourself off from ever experiencing life to the fullest, because you're not living in the present. In fact, when you're that numb, you're not really living at all. Your mind is focused on the future, on what *may* happen if you allow yourself to do such and such, so you're sacrificing the present for something that may never happen in the future.

Put In Your Application for Recovery

If you want to get a job, you have to apply. If it's a really great job and you really want it, you might be worried that you won't get it. In fact, you might talk yourself out of even applying. If you don't apply, you won't risk being disappointed, right? But if you don't apply, you also won't stand a chance of getting the job, and you'll never know if you would have gotten it.

Three Tries and You're In!

I want you to take a trip with me for a moment back to sixth grade. Do you remember the science fair projects your teachers made you do? Which one was your favorite? Mine was definitely the exploding volcano. One of the main purposes of these projects was to learn the scientific method:

1. Ask a question.
2. Do the research.
3. Construct a hypothesis.
4. Test your hypothesis with an experiment.
5. Analyze your results.
6. Report your conclusion.

And when you were testing your hypothesis, your teacher probably told you to do your experiment three times to make sure your results were accurate.

When the people I work with try something new (or take a risk), I always ask them to give the activity three tries, just as we learned to do with the scientific method.

Do it once and you'll know that you can get through it. It might be very painful, but see, you did it!

Try it again and it might not be as scary—it might be, but then again, maybe it won't.

By the third time it will be easier still, and you'll realize that you'll be able to keep on doing it.

It's uncomfortable applying for a job—filling out the application, going through the interview process, waiting to find out if you've been accepted. And that's true of almost anything you want in life. You've got to go through the discomfort in order to achieve. But if you deny yourself the chance of achieving, you'll actually be hurting—not protecting—yourself. You may avoid the pain, but you'll also deny yourself the good that might have come your way. So, don't deny yourself the chance to get healthy; take a risk, put in your application for recovery and commit to doing whatever it takes to succeed.

Sinkies and Floaties — What Pulls You Down and What Gets You Through?

When you start to do something different, such as working on your recovery, it can feel very lonely, and you're going to need some support. Are you familiar with those inflatable armbands called floaties that little kids wear in the pool? When you first started to get involved with your eating disorder, there might have been some triggering event in your life, large or small, that was trying to sink you, and your eating disorder was what you believed kept you afloat. It gave you something to focus on so that you didn't have to think about whatever it was that you needed to block out. But very quickly, the thing that had been helping you to keep your head above water started to pull you under. Your eating disorder transformed into a sinkie.

But you do have floaties — we all do. Imagine that you're wearing a pair of floaties on your arms. Take a moment to visualize what they would look like. You can decorate them any way you want. Mine would have bright yellow lightning bolts to remind me of the power I reclaimed from my eating disorder, but yours might have beautiful pink roses to remind you of how beautiful life is, or even images of loved ones to remind you of all the people who want you to recover and believe that you can.

Floaties are the people who support us, be they family members, members of a support group, a good friend or a significant other. Floaties are those people, places or things that help keep us afloat when we're inevitably feeling the force that's trying to push us down. Floaties are the things that give us pleasure in life—the things that make us smile. What makes you smile? Is it an animal, a good book, a song, sitting on the beach, working in the garden, spending time with family and friends? Those are all floaties.

Floaties are those people, places or things that help keep us afloat when we're inevitably feeling the force that's trying to push us down. Floaties are the things that give us pleasure in life—the things that make us smile.

When you're on an even keel and life is smooth sailing, you'll begin to notice the little everyday miracles in your life—your dog wagging his tail when he's asleep, the little birds flying down the highway that seem to be following your car, a great song, a beautiful sunrise.

Here are the things that make me smile:

- My dog, Sammie, cocking his head as if he is listening when I am speaking to him
- My cat, Leela, jumping straight up in the air when she gets spooked
- My mother's smile
- My husband Max's "little boy" belly laugh or the silly songs he makes up and sings around the house
- The faces of the brave and inspiring women in my Monday Night Support Group
- A special "helllllooooo" at the beginning of a phone conversation
- The amazing friends in my life that I am so lucky to have
- A Sale sign in the window of my favorite store

When you notice the things that make you smile, write them down. Create your own smile list. These will be your floaties so that when a sinkie comes along and tries to drag you under—when you're having one of those black-crayon days—you can pull out your list and remind yourself of all the good and supportive things in your life.

Take hold of the real floaties in your life.
Trust in yourself and your support system.
Do not let yourself be fooled by your
eating disorder again.

Don't Fall for the Bait and Switch

Initially, your eating disorder gave you a sense of control, but in reality it was a false sense of control. It sucked you in like an advertising come-on and then, when you were hooked, it turned around and started to control you. It convinced you it was there to save you, to help keep you safe, but in reality it was doing just the opposite.

Take hold of the real floaties in your life. Trust in yourself and your support system. Do not let yourself be fooled by your eating disorder again.

PS: Your eating disorder may still sometimes try to disguise itself as a floatie. But even if it's wearing a fancy costume and is desperately trying to convince you that it is there to keep you afloat, it is still, beneath that disguise, your eating disorder. So don't be fooled! Let it go, let it sink to the bottom and make sure that your pool drain is open to suck it up.

Chapter Four

KICKING OFF THE OTHER SHOE

The greatest barrier to success is the fear of failure.
—Sven-Göran Eriksson,
renowned Swedish football (soccer) manager

You're about to start the recovery process. You're holding tight to your white crayon, and you're fully committed to taking care of yourself. But you're very, very afraid; you've been living in a black-and-white world for so long that you assume this recovery thing is going to be either all good (top drawer), or all bad (bottom drawer). You can't imagine anything in between, so when you trip up, which almost always happens during the recovery process, you crash, and you figure that since you're failing anyway, you might just as well kick off that other shoe and get it over with.

We have all heard the popular saying "waiting for the other shoe to drop." Well, if you are anything like I was during my battle with my eating disorder and even in the early years of recovery, you're probably so afraid of being hurt, happy, sad, succeeding or failing, or feeling anything at all that you're likely to kick off the other shoe before it has a chance to fall on its own. I know I did that because I really thought it was a way for me to control the outcome. It took me a long time to figure out that contrary to what I believed, kicking off the other shoe is a self-fulfilling prophecy that ensures you won't succeed.

You're probably so afraid of being hurt, happy, sad, succeeding or failing, or feeling anything at all that you're likely to kick off the other shoe before it has a chance to fall on its own.

For years I had so little self-love that I couldn't imagine why anyone else would be friends with me, let alone love me. I didn't think I deserved that love, and to my mind, being in a romantic relationship was simply not in the cards. Since I didn't believe anyone could love me, I assumed that anyone who came close to me would wind up hurting me in the end.

When I started dating Max, the amazing man who would become my husband, I assumed I'd wind up being hurt, and I couldn't let that happen because I knew the pain I'd feel if I allowed him to hurt me would be much worse than the pain I'd feel if I hurt myself. I was also convinced that once he got to know me, he would be so turned off by my story and my battle that he would inevitably run as fast as he could in the other direction. So what did I do? Just about everything in my power to push him away. I never let myself sit still and just be with him. I kept constantly busy and made sure I did every-thing *but* spend time with him. And even when we *were* spending time together, I was very wary of letting him get to know the real me. I knew that I simply couldn't endure the pain of allowing myself to let him in and then getting hurt. I thought that if I let down my guard and let him get close, he might leave and I would be heartbroken. At least if I did it to myself, I'd be in control of the outcome and wouldn't hurt as much (or so I'd convinced myself). Luckily for me, Max just wouldn't let me push him away. He kept on telling me that although I didn't feel I was worth it, he thought I was worth fighting for.

We've already talked about the fact that however negative the behaviors, your eating disorder has been providing you with a kind of safe haven. When you're in the midst of an eating disorder, you know that if you do A, the outcome will be B. And even though that kind of thinking is incredibly self-limiting, it is also perversely comforting.

For years I had so little self-love that I couldn't imagine why anyone else would be friends with me, let alone love me. I didn't think I deserved that love.

So let me ask you this: What would happen if, just once, you didn't kick off that other shoe? What if you got a shoe that fit so well it didn't come off? Or what if you kept both feet firmly planted on the ground so that it couldn't come off? Realistically, recovery is about white-knuckling through your fear and having faith that the shoe won't necessarily come off. Maybe it will, but maybe it won't. The only certainty is that if you kick it off, it's never going to land in a good place. You may know where it's going to land, but that landing spot will be a place of negativity. And if the shoe does come off on its own, you can always go out and buy another, better-fitting pair—that's also your choice.

No, the Sky Isn't Purple

If I try to tell you that the sky is purple, at first you're going to look up, see that it's blue and tell me I'm nuts. But if I keep telling you over and over, day after day, that the sky is purple, and if I sound absolutely certain of what I'm saying, eventually you'll start to question yourself. You'll begin to think maybe you're the one who's nuts, and that even though it looks blue to you, the sky really is purple. Over time, you may even start to see the sky as purple. That's what your negative voice has been doing to you for so long. It keeps telling you that you're not good enough, you're undeserving (well, you get the point—no need to let the negative voice have any more space on this page), to the point where you internalize that voice and what it's been telling you becomes your perceived reality.

Your negative voice has been telling you that you're not good enough, you're undeserving, to the point where you internalize that message and it becomes your perceived reality.

Once that negativity becomes your reality, it's impossible to believe that anything good could possibly come your way. So you start to build a protective wall around yourself. You have a hard time even being with friends and family; you're afraid to open yourself up to anyone, because if you did, you'd be vulnerable. Instead of thinking, *Hey, maybe I could make a really good friend here and add another floatie to my support system,* you automatically think, *How is this person going to hurt me? When is this person going to leave?* Instead of putting yourself out there and waiting to see what happens, you write the final chapter of your own book. In fact, you are so focused on the negative and so convinced that the eating disorder is your protector, you can't even see a real floatie when it's right there in front of you, begging to be let in.

Imagine that you listen to a message on your answering machine and decide that you hear something negative in the caller's voice. You immediately start to imagine what could be wrong, what you could possibly have done to elicit that negativity, and before you ever return the call, you've written an entire epic novel in your head about what you did wrong to make that person angry (because, of course, your negative voice has convinced you that it is all your fault the person is angry). You know you need to return your friend's call, but you're so afraid of confrontation that you let a few days go by before you pick up the phone. When you finally do work up the courage and return the call, the first thing you say is, "Are you okay? Did I do something to upset you? I'm so sorry if I hurt you in any way." Just by saying those words, you're creating a wall between yourself and the other person—even though it's highly likely that his or her anger was a figment of your imagination or had nothing at all to do with you. More than likely, your friend won't even know what you're talking about.

As time goes on, you keep building your protective wall higher and higher, because you believe you're about to be attacked and wounded by a hostile army. Realistically, however, when you build such a high wall, you may keep the bad out, but you also keep out the good. Even if you realize there may be some folks out there who aren't out to hurt you, whom you really do like and want to know better, the wall you've built is so strong and so tall that there's no way you can climb over it or create an opening to let them in.

CHAPTER

Knocking Down the Wall

How do you start to knock down that wall? First of all, you need to understand that you built your wall out of fear. You built it out of your own negative thoughts. I'm not saying it's your fault. You were trying to feel better, trying to protect yourself. It was not something you did consciously by waking up one morning and saying, "I think I'm terrible and no one will want me or love me, so I will build a wall to keep everyone out." But build it you did, and the only way to dismantle it is to take a few risks and start to think more positively. Easier said than done, you say? Absolutely. But you can do it.

Your eating disorder and the negative thoughts and behaviors surrounding it may have been helping you to survive, but life is about giving yourself the chance to thrive, not just survive.

Your eating disorder and the negative thoughts and behaviors surrounding it may have been helping you to survive, but that's not what life should be about. Life is about giving yourself the chance to thrive, not just survive. Repeat after me: "I, [insert your name], deserve to thrive, not just survive." Yes, sometimes, even if you don't kick it off, the other shoe will drop. Life is not always bunnies and rainbows and sunshine! But remember, if you don't give yourself the chance to fail, you'll never have the opportunity to succeed and have new, amazing and exciting experiences.

Start by getting just one leg over that wall. It's not going to be easy because you've done a really good job of building it in the first place. But it's definitely worth the effort. So, you put a leg over the wall and open up to one person. Maybe that person is going to be the best friend you could ever have in the whole, entire world—someone who will literally go the extra mile for you, hold your hand every step of the way and be there through thick and thin. That's your top-drawer scenario. Or maybe you'll discover that the person you open up to fulfills every negative thought you've ever had about allowing yourself to open up to people. That's your bottom-drawer scenario. But more likely you'll make a good friend, someone you can talk to and who will be there when you need an extra boost without being totally involved in every moment of your life. That's living in the middle drawer—a very healthy place to be. And keep in mind that your circle of friends may change over time as you continue your journey to recovery.

Remember when we talked about taking the risk of applying for a job? Not putting in that application is a paradigmatic example of what it means to kick off the other shoe and write the end of the book before you've ever given the plotline a chance to develop. What's the best thing that could happen if you applied for the job? Not only would you get the job, but you could be promoted to CEO, enjoy every perk that goes along with the job, become recognized throughout the world and earn a seven-figure salary. Top-, top-drawer! And, worst-case scenario, you could be told you weren't qualified and you wouldn't get the job. Maybe your prospective employer would even ask you why you bothered to apply. That's definitely bottom-drawer. Or, you'd get the job, be given the usual three months' probation and have to work hard to prove yourself to your new employer. You'd complete your work on time, listen to critical feedback and try your best. Now, it's possible that at the end of the three months you'd be told it wasn't working out. But equally, if not much more likely, you'd finish your probation period and settle into your new position. There will be days you love your new job, there will be days you really do not like your new job, but most days would be middle-drawer okay.

Don't Start Out as a Downer

There isn't anyone in the world who can't make her/himself crazy by thinking of all the negative what-ifs that are (probably) never going to happen. But when you're struggling with an eating disorder and caught up in black-and-white thinking, you're more vulnerable than most other people to getting caught up in that worst-possible-scenario way of thinking.

When I was caught up in my own negative thoughts, I was constantly looking around me and believing that everyone else was smarter, braver, more attractive, a better friend, more charming—simply better in every way than I was.

When we were discussing this in group not too long ago, one of the women raised her hand and told the group that she had a son with epilepsy who was going to be starting a new school very soon. She was going to have to talk to his teachers and explain his condition, and that was causing her a lot of stress because she just *knew* that they wouldn't understand. She was convinced that the teachers wouldn't know what to do if he had a seizure, they might not be familiar with the medical protocol and just by sending him to school she'd be putting his life in danger. By the time she was done, she'd already stuffed herself into the bottom drawer, pulled it shut after her and locked it from the inside with a dead bolt. She'd forcefully kicked off the other shoe before it had a chance to fall on its own.

When I was caught up in my own negative thoughts, I was constantly looking around me and believing that everyone else was smarter, braver, more attractive, a better friend, more charming—simply better in every way than I was. In my own mind, I was always the worst of the worst, the lowest of the low. For a long time I believed that I was the only person who felt that way. It didn't occur to me that other people could actually feel as bad about themselves as I did about myself. Looking back on that time now, it's amazing how distorted the view from my negative-colored glasses really was.

By kicking off the other shoe, you're making certain you're right, because you're making sure that the situation turns out the way you were afraid it would—badly.

In truth, I had no idea what was going on in the lives of those other people. I just made up their stories in my own head, whether or not they had anything to do with reality. I truly believed that I was the one person on earth who wouldn't ever get better, that I wouldn't be good enough to do it. And so, for the longest time, I kept kicking off that other shoe so that I could be certain the story I was telling myself would come true.

By kicking off the other shoe, you're making certain you're right, because you're making sure that the situation (whatever it is) turns out the way you were afraid it would—badly. And then, when it does end badly, you can say, "See, I told you so." But would you really, truly, rather be right than give yourself the chance to be happy? I think they call that self-sabotage.

You've Got to Be in It to Win It

That slogan is just as applicable to your recovery as it was to the New York Lottery.

Picture this scenario: you're terrified of going to the supermarket, where you'll be surrounded by triggering foods, and you're certain that everyone will stare at you because they know there's something going on with you.

But you gather up your courage, take the risk and go to the store. You take a shopping cart and start walking down the aisle. One of the wheels on the cart is squeaking, and you're mentally cursing it for drawing attention to you. But you tell yourself you can do this. You're going to be okay. You make your selections and get in line at the checkout counter. Then, just as you get up to the cashier and start to take the first item out of your cart, lights start to flash, bells and whistles go off. You're informed that you're the millionth customer and you've just won an enormous prize package that includes an all-expenses-paid trip to the destination of your choice anywhere in the world. Top-drawer!

What are the odds of that happening? Not great. But sometimes the thing you're most afraid of turns out to end better than you could ever have imagined. I can tell you that's absolutely true of my life in recovery. Sometimes surprise endings are happy endings. But if you don't take the risk, you'll never put yourself in the running for the prize. You've got to be in it to win it! And sometimes you'll take the risk and the result is simply neutral—middle-drawer. You'll do your shopping, check out and drive home without any incident, either good or bad. That, too, will be an accomplishment.

And the Real Secret Is…

If there's one secret a lot of people know that those of us battling an eating disorder might find hard to believe, it is the concept that you can fail and it won't be the end of the world. What they understand is that everything in the world isn't always black-and-white and that it's absolutely okay to be okay. That's a really important, not-so-secret secret.

Everything in the world isn't always black-and-white. It's absolutely okay to be okay.

There are a lot of negative words associated with *okay*—*boring, not good enough, mediocre, dull*. But *okay* is also calm, peaceful, serene. For those of us who have been struggling for a while, it might be difficult to imagine what it feels like to be calm. I like to ask the people in my groups to visualize themselves floating on a big inner tube in a lake and being totally relaxed. The water is totally still—not even a ripple. They are not allowed to focus on what they look like in the tube, just on their environment. We did this exercise not too long ago, and I had to laugh when one woman immediately raised her hand and asked, "You want me to be calm, but what about the sharks?" Her negative response was an absolute knee-jerk reaction to the very idea that she could be okay. Anyone can turn any kind of positive into a negative, but realistically sharks don't swim in lakes. She was just kicking off the other shoe so that she wouldn't have to take the risk of allowing herself to just be okay. Not top-drawer, not bottom-drawer, just staying on an even keel and being somewhere in the middle.

All I'm asking is that you take that risk. Find a floatie, put on your protective gear and keep that shoe on for just a few minutes longer. I know it's scary, but you can do it. If it does fall of its own accord, it may actually fall in a good place—and maybe it will just stay on. Sometimes the outcome will be great, sometimes it will be painful, but most of the time it will be okay. The more you take the risk of not kicking off that shoe, the more empowered you will be to do it again. The law of averages says that if you keep it on, you'll experience more positive outcomes than if you keep kicking it off. You'll be letting some good into your life, and you deserve to feel good.

All I'm asking is that you take that risk.
Find a floatie, put on your protective gear and
keep that shoe on for just a few minutes longer.

If recovery were easy, everyone would be doing it right away; no one would hesitate or struggle. If it were so easy to feel good about yourself, everyone would be feeling good about themselves all the time. But the truth is, it's the easiest thing in the world for human beings to sabotage themselves, and we're all human. Make a commitment to yourself and your health. Commit to stopping the self-sabotage. It won't happen overnight, but with commitment you can do this. It's worth it, and you deserve it.

One of the most difficult things I have done during the past nine years of my recovery was watch one of one my closest friends relapse and start battling her eating disorder all over again. Even though I knew what I was supposed to say and how I was supposed to act, this was someone I cared about deeply, and all I really wanted to do was throw my arms around her and make it go away. Of course, I couldn't do that. All I could do was support her until she was ready to ask for help. Thankfully, Jasmine did ask for help. She received the treatment she needed and has become a role model to other women in treatment. Four years later, she is not only surviving but thriving. She has graduated from a doctoral program, gotten married and had a healthy baby girl. She is recovered from her eating disorder and is living proof that recovery is worth it.

I suffered from anorexia and bulimia for almost eight years. While in the past I tended to focus on everything I lost because of my eating disorder, I've now been able to turn my experience into something more positive. Although I suffered a tremendous amount of pain when I was struggling with my disorder, I also grew stronger and gained a sense of direction during my healing process.

Growing up, I did gymnastics for several years and was naturally petite. After I quit gymnastics, however, I began to go through puberty, and while my weight increased, my height remained the same. It was also about this time that I entered a competitive arts school. Never having been a person who works extremely well under pressure, I didn't think that I measured up to my peers and I didn't believe I deserved to be in the school. I was constantly comparing my abilities, my grades and my body to those of other people, judging myself unworthy and feeling depressed.

It's hard to pinpoint exactly when my eating disorder began, but shortly after entering the arts school, I lost someone who had been a mother figure to me for ten years. I didn't attend her funeral, and for years afterward I lived with the guilt of missing it and of pushing her away as I grew older. The emptiness I felt as a result of her loss remained with me for years. I had difficulty expressing those feelings and was sinking deeper and deeper into depression.

About a year after her death, I tried to take control of my life by restricting my food intake. I started by skipping meals, which ultimately led to days of fasting. In eleventh grade I began to abuse laxatives and spent quite a bit of time doubled over on the floor during classes. Ironically, the one thing that had given me a sense of control (my eating disorder) became the very thing that spiraled out of my control.

> The one thing that had given me a sense of control became the very thing that spiraled out of my control.

In retrospect, I realize that I no doubt had a genetic predisposition to developing an eating disorder. My mother was also anorexic, and my grandmother most likely had some type of eating disorder, but the stress and guilt I was experiencing were the triggers that set mine in motion.

At first, no one addressed my weight loss, which led me to believe it wasn't noticeable. I strove to lose more and practically lived on the scale. The scale served as a sanctuary, yet it could also be a tormentor. I felt proud of my motivation and accomplishment when I lost a pound, and I punished myself if I didn't. While I was aware that I had some kind of a problem, I didn't realize its severity and was not ready to seek help.

After graduating high school, I entered a local university because I was afraid to move out of my parents' home. I was becoming more and more depressed, unable to focus or concentrate, and even passing out from time to time. I knew I was going to crash at some point, but I didn't know how fast it would happen. Early in the first semester of my freshman year, I received a letter from an old friend from high school, who confronted me about having an eating disorder. She said that several people had wanted to contact my parents but were afraid I'd be upset with them.

After several years of carrying this secret alone, I broke down and told her I was struggling with food issues. My friend then told me that there was an eating disorder screening at my university and said she would go with me.

I was fortunate to meet a wonderful person at the screening, a woman who had struggled with an eating disorder herself. Years later, she still served as a mentor, giving me strength, hope and love. She took me to the counseling center, where, quite frankly, I manipulated and lied to my therapist for several months. I was leading a double life, smiling in public and breaking down in private.

> I was leading a double life, smiling in public and breaking down in private.

At this point, I knew I was very sick. My body was weak and I had difficulty concentrating, walking, even speaking. My blood tests were abnormal, my fingernails were purple, and I was constantly in pain. As I was leaving my therapy session one day, I was literally unable to hold myself up and fell to the floor. My therapist and her supervisor said that I needed to tell my mother about my eating disorder immediately. If I didn't tell my parents, they said, I would be involuntarily committed to the hospital.

I felt betrayed and backed into a corner, but the scare tactic worked. Feeling exposed, ashamed and terrified, I told my mother that I had an eating disorder. After that, I immediately entered therapy with an eating disorder specialist, which was quite possibly one of the worst experiences in my life. It quickly became apparent that my therapist was still active in her own eating disorder and that it was affecting her work. She complained of low blood sugar, walked out of group sessions to tend to personal problems and encouraged us to have liposuction and use diet pills.

My physician was also monitoring me closely, and when my weekly weigh-in showed that I wasn't adhering to my contract to maintain a particular weight, I admitted that I was using laxatives again. My lab work also showed several abnormalities, and, in addition, I was severely dehydrated. The doctor informed me that we would have to discuss treatment options—including an inpatient facility—with my mother, or else she would be forced to terminate treatment with me.

My parents fought long and hard with their insurance company to cover my treatment as an inpatient at an eating disorder facility. Looking back on the situation, I realize now that I needed to be there because I didn't care if I lived or died. However, at the time, I was furious that people were trying to take away my "friend," the eating disorder.

While my parents were still fighting to get me the help I needed, I began to go on bingeing and purging episodes with other people, which left me feeling disgusted, helpless and hopeless. After my mother informed the insurance company that I was going to kill myself, they finally approved two days in a treatment facility, which caused me to feel extremely pressured to cure myself in what was clearly an unrealistic time frame.

In the end, I was very fortunate that my parents were able to find the money for me to remain at the treatment facility for as long as necessary. I stayed almost three months, during which time I gathered coping tools, gained a better understanding of myself and worked with a good therapist.

Recovery was a roller-coaster ride, and I suffered several relapses after being released. However, several years later I had made tremendous progress in my recovery and entered a doctoral program in clinical psychology. While I still had lingering concerns about the pressures I would face in such a program, I pushed them away and moved forward with my dream, which was to work with children with disabilities.

During my third year in graduate school, I began to have several setbacks. I once again became focused on my weight and body, and started struggling with feelings of depression. I felt myself crashing shortly before defending my dissertation and reentered an eating disorder facility.

For once, I was not afraid of what the future held or even of letting go of my eating disorder. I had experienced periods of being symptom free, and I knew how incredible life could be.

This time I was motivated to change. I stayed for about thirty days before my insurance benefits ran out, and I know I was fortunate to have stayed that long. Before being discharged, I was told that I had inspired many of the other patients there. I do not say this to brag but because of how shocked I was to hear that! How could someone who had been so depressed and hopeless for years and years become an inspiration to other people?

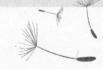

For once, I was not afraid of what the future held or even of letting go of my eating disorder. I had experienced periods of being symptom free, and I knew how incredible life could be.

....

I consider myself 100 percent recovered and cannot imagine ever going back to my eating disorder.

....

At this time, I have been completely symptom free for four years. Incredibly, I am now a doctor of psychology, a wife and a mother. I consider myself 100 percent recovered and cannot imagine ever going back to my eating disorder. I want to be a role model for my daughter, and I want to break the cycle of eating disorders in my family. I accept the challenges life brings, and I allow myself to feel everything I should. I am in a place I never thought I would be, and I would not change it for the world.

Chapter Five

FROM RECOVERING TO RECOVERED—IT'S A PROCESS

To get through the hardest journey we need take only

one step at a time, but we must keep on stepping.

—CHINESE PROVERB

FOR A LONG TIME AFTER I STARTED the recovery process, I told people I was "recovering" from my eating disorder. In fact, I'd always been told that some aspect of my eating disorder—whether it was a distorted body image, lack of self-esteem or not having a strong and powerful voice—would always be with me. In addition, when I first chose recovery, I wasn't really ready to face a world in which my eating disorder would no longer be part of my life—a world in which I was "recovered." Getting to the place where I would be recovered felt impossible, like something I wouldn't be able to accomplish. And, truth be told, I found some degree of comfort in the idea that some part of my eating disorder would always be a part of my life. I wasn't ready to give that up entirely. While I could face the prospect of recovering, being recovered was just too scary for me, too final.

How Long Can You Be Recovering?

For years, when I shared my story in schools or in groups, I would say, "It's been five years [or six years or eight years] that I've been recovering from my eating disorder. Some aspect of it will always be with me." I truly thought that was the right thing to tell people. I thought I was being open and honest. I came from the school of thought that believed I would always be fighting some sort of battle (even if it was a small one).

While I could face the prospect of recovering, being recovered was just too scary for me, too final.

Then one day, as I was getting ready to start a group, I asked each of the attendees to tell the rest of us who she was, why she was there and a little bit about her experience. To start things off, I said, "My name is Johanna, and I've been recovering from my eating disorder for the past eight years." The minute those words were out of my mouth, I saw a few faces fall and realized that I immediately needed to talk about their reaction. "Okay," I said. "Let's talk about what's going on here."

"It sounds like it's never going to go away," one woman replied. "It sounds as if it's always going to be a battle. It's always going to be in the forefront of my mind. I really don't know if I'll be able to fight this fight for the rest of my life."

*Having an eating disorder was no
longer my identity. A lightbulb went on.
I, Johanna Kandel, was recovered.*

Hearing those words, believe it or not, caused me to take a step back and really examine where I was in my own recovery. I realized then that I was no longer living my life for my eating disorder. It wasn't the first thing I thought about when I woke up in the morning, the last thing I thought about at night, and it wasn't every thought in between. Having an eating disorder was no longer my identity. A lightbulb went on. I, Johanna Kandel, was recovered. Maybe I was never going to run down the street naked, yelling, "Look at me. I am so fabulous" (how many women would?), but I had come to a place where I'd become friends with and respected my self and my body. Me, friends with my body? Not in this lifetime, or so I had thought! But boy, was I wrong. When I started my journey, I would never have thought I would ever get to the place I am at now.

*I had come to a place where I'd become
friends with and respected my self and my body.*

I realized that telling people I'd been recovering for eight years was not only inaccurate, but it was also unhelpful. When you choose to embark on a radical life change, you know it's going to be tough for a while. If you're assured that it will get easier and eventually it won't be very difficult at all, you'll know there's a light at the end of the tunnel, and just knowing that can be enough to keep you going. But if you think it will be a never-ending, monumental battle, you might just give up before you've ever begun. I want to encourage you with all of my being to fight the fight, take those chances and embark on one of the most worthwhile journeys of all—the journey to yourself and recovery.

Each Moment Is a New Opportunity

What was it that made you choose recovery? Sometimes life change starts with just opening the door a crack and catching a glimpse of what's on the other side. The first time you did that, you might have taken a peek and then run to hide under the covers. The second time maybe you opened the door a bit wider, stood there a bit longer and got a better look. And then maybe you took a step outside and lingered long enough to breathe the fresh air. Gradually you'll be able to walk through that door and keep on going. That's how recovery happens—a glimmer at a time. It's a process, and you can do it.

Fight the fight, take those chances and embark on one of the most worthwhile journeys of all—the journey to yourself and recovery.

I'm not going to lie; starting the recovery process is hard. Each step you take on the path to recovery will lead you to a fork in the road. And each time you get to another fork, you'll have to make a decision about which way to go. Will you do the next right thing for yourself and your health, or will you make a self-sabotaging choice? The negative, eating disorder voice in your head will be arguing with your healthy voice about which way to go, and in the beginning your eating disorder voice will be really loud, while your healthy voice may be no louder than a whisper. You may encounter any number of those small choices in the course of a given day. Constantly engaging in that kind of battle is exhausting. If you thought it was going to be like that forever, I wouldn't blame you for giving up. But it won't be. You have to have faith. You will succeed.

Take It One Meal at a Time

Very often people will make healthy choices for a meal, a day or two or three, and then they'll suddenly realize what they've been doing, and it will become so overwhelming that they respond by acting out or giving in to their eating disorder.

What I tell people is that a day is a day, a meal is a meal, a moment is a moment. Don't let the fact that you did well at breakfast or lunch or for one whole day overwhelm you into worrying that you have to live up to some standard you've established for yourself. Pat yourself on the back for your healthy behavior and move on to the next moment, and then the next moment after that. Leave each meal behind when you leave the table. Start afresh with the next meal. Know what you can do in the moment. Stop thinking about next week, next month, next year. Concentrate on the now, and if you do happen to slip at one meal, pick yourself up and leave it behind. Move on. You have the power to make a different choice the next time. It really is about taking it one moment at a time.

A day is a day, a meal is a meal,
a moment is a moment.

Think of me as a scout who's traveled that path ahead of you and returned with news of what lies down the road. Luckily, the forecast is good. At first you might feel as if you're fighting an uphill battle; your eating disorder voice will have a large army equipped with heavy-duty weapons, while you'll have just one or two part-time soldiers on your healthy side. It's not going to seem like a fair fight. But what you'll discover is that with each good decision you make, you'll be adding another loyal soldier to your army. Gradually your positive, healthy voice will become stronger and louder until it's actually out-shouting your eating disorder voice. Imagine that your healthy voice has a bull-horn turned up to the loudest setting, and your eating disorder/negative voice can barely be heard. After a while, you won't even need the bullhorn anymore.

Gradually your positive, healthy voice will become stronger and louder until it's actually outshouting your eating disorder voice.

But remember that this is a journey, and the topography won't always be smooth. Some days you'll be in the fast lane, moving full speed ahead. But some days you'll hit a speed bump or two, and some days you'll be caught in a traffic jam and not moving at all. The interesting thing about the road to recovery, however, is that even when you're standing still, you're actually moving forward just because you're not moving backward. You're still farther along than you were when you started out; you're getting stronger, and you're consolidating your gains. In fact, that is part of learning to be okay—not speeding ahead, not going backward, just being okay.

On the road to recovery, even when you're standing still, you're actually moving forward. You're still farther along than you were when you started out; you're getting stronger, and you're consolidating your gains.

One way I found to remind myself of how far I'd come was to write myself a letter when I was doing the next right thing and feeling strong in my recovery. Then, on those inevitable days when I was feeling overwhelmed and defeated by my eating disorder and the recovery process, I had proof that I'd had good days and was succeeding. Here's one of the letters I wrote to remind myself of the great day I'd had:

Dear Johanna,

Today was a great day. I feel really strong and powerful. I can honestly say that I was able to truly take care of myself. I am so proud! Yippee! I was able to smile, laugh and even tell my coworker that the comment she made about a crazy new diet was triggering and not healthy for her or for me. Yay! My first boundary,

I stood up for myself and boy, did it feel good. Although I was scared, I knew I had to use my voice. And guess what? It worked! It felt so good, and I feel so strong right now. Today is proof that if I keep on putting one foot in front of the other, I will reach my goal. I know that my path has been long and at times arduous; I just need to remember to have faith and trust in the recovery process.

Now, in case you are reading this and having a bad day, please know that you are strong, capable and willing. You have already overcome so much, and I am so proud of you. This letter is a reminder that although every day may not have been fantastic, you have had amazing days, too, and there will be more to come. You can do this!

You deserve all the happiness and health in the world. It's not going to be perfect, but you are going to make it through, and it's going to be so worth it! It is so important for you to continue your journey.

So, next time you feel beaten down or defeated about your recovery, remember how you felt today (how I feel right now). You should have the utmost faith in yourself, because you know what? You deserve to be happy and healthy. You deserve to live your life to the fullest. And today is proof of that. So keep your head up, dust yourself off and keep on moving.

Lots of love,

Johanna

PS: I think you are fabulous! Do not forget it.

Why Does It Have to Be So Hard?

Change is always hard, even when you know it's something you really want to do. No matter how long you've been struggling with your eating disorder, it's become what you know, it's familiar, it's second nature, and, above all, it's provided you with a false sense of safety. However negative your behaviors might have been, they were providing you with something you needed. The behaviors felt like floaties because they and their outcomes were predictable, even though they were dragging you down.

In fact, you may feel as if your eating disorder has been what's defined you; without it you'll need to begin to asking yourself who you are. The idea that you're going to have to redefine yourself is scary, and that's why it's so hard. What's so scary about recovery for you? I encourage you to take a moment and make a list of what it is about the recovery process that's really, really scary for you. When I've done this exercise with my groups, I've heard answers like the following:

- I will have to figure out what I like and what I don't like.
- I am going to have to deal with my emotions.
- I am going to have to feel again. Ugh!
- I am going to have to confront people and use my voice.
- I am going to have to deal with intimacy.

Establish a Special Savings Account

Each positive step you take, no matter how small, is like putting money in the bank (*cha-ching*)! The only difference is that unlike a bank account, when you put money in your "recovery account," it stays there forever. The balance will never be diminished because what's deposited can never be withdrawn. As you begin to make deposits in your account, keep a record, like the ledger in your savings book. As you see your balance grow, you'll discover how much you've already invested in your recovery, and you'll build the confidence and momentum you need to keep moving forward. You can always go back and enjoy the investments you've already made, and you'll also feel good about the fact that your deposits will continue to grow.

PS: Investing in your recovery promises a million percent return rate!

Among all these fears, the two I hear most often are: *I may find out that I don't like who I am without my eating disorder* and *I'm afraid I might get to the end of the journey and realize that recovery really wasn't worth it.* Well, guess what? It *is* worth it! Walking through my own fears (white-knuckling it at times) was a challenge, but I can tell you that there is no doubt about it—it was and is the best thing I have ever done. And honestly, I have never heard anyone else say that it wasn't worth it, either.

Walking through my own fears was a challenge, but I can tell you that there is no doubt about it— it was and is the best thing I have ever done.

Nothing Is Written in Indelible Ink

When it comes to facing the fear of learning who you are, I like to remind people that no one is asking you to become someone else. When you set out on a journey you take yourself with you, and although the journey may be transformational, the person you wind up with is (drumroll, please) still you. The second thing I tell them is that no one's expecting them to answer all those big questions all at once. No one is expecting you to write an epic, one-thousand-page autobiography that contains every detail about your likes and dislikes the minute you enter recovery—or ever, for that matter!

Get out a pencil with a really big eraser and start writing down what you like and what you don't. What colors do you like? What activities? What books, movies, music, colors, clothing, fabrics? The list can be as long or as short as you make it. You may find that starting out you have no idea what you like or dislike, because you've been so defined by your eating disorder that you haven't even thought about the choices you might make if it were no longer the defining characteristic of your life. Choice may never have seemed like an option to you, but when you get past your eating disorder you do have options. Remember that this is a journey, and you may find out that what you like today, or the choices you make today, are not the same as what you'll like or choose two weeks or two months from now.

Open up your crayon box again, pick out a color and try it to see if you like it. Maybe you'll discover that you love the cerise crayon. But maybe two weeks later you'll decide you don't really like that one, after all. That's the beauty of writing in pencil and having a big eraser. You can always change your mind. The point is that you do get to choose. You hold that power now and you will hold that power forever, so long as you don't ever choose to give it away.

If you were writing with indelible ink, you'd always be afraid that you'd be stuck with the choices you made, but you're not. We don't write with indelible ink anymore. We use computers, which allow us to change our minds, cut and paste, and change things around to our hearts' content. Your eating disorder wrote in indelible ink and saw the world in black-and-white; you don't have to. Realizing that is going to be like removing a giant brick from your backpack; it will be a huge weight lifted from your shoulders.

And, even more exciting, you'll probably start to find that you like different things on different days! Maybe one day you'll like staying home alone with a good book. On another day you might want to meet up with friends and go to a movie. One day you might want to put on your most colorful outfit and a really bright red lipstick, and tomorrow you'll declare a makeup-free, jeans-and-sneakers day. That's what happens when you get away from thinking only in black-and-white. You realize that your choices are endless and that you've been preventing yourself from experiencing the full spectrum of colors life has to offer. Once you feel comfortable with that idea, you will have a tremendous sense of freedom. It's out there for you, and you deserve it!

Remember—You're Still You

Yes, I know, I've been telling you how transforming this journey will be, but in all honesty I have to point out that even transformed, you're still going to be you. Even when you're recovered, you're not going to become a totally different person. Think of your healthy self as a long-lost friend. There is something vaguely familiar about this old friend, but you still need to take time to learn what she's been up to since the last time you saw her. You owe it to yourself and your friend to take the time to get to know her again. I suspect you will really like her if you truly get to know her.

Remember that there is an underlying genetic component to the reason you developed an eating disorder and someone else, given a similar set of circumstances, did not. Something about our makeups made us more vulnerable than the next person to developing an eating disorder, and that hasn't changed. If you were a perfectionist, if you had obsessive-compulsive tendencies, those tendencies will still be there. Everything doesn't change. The big, all-important difference is that once you're aware of them, you can choose to deal with them in a healthier, more positive way. They no longer need to run your life.

I know I'm a perfectionist. When I was in college I would go home after class and copy my notes so that they'd be neater, even though I was the only person who would ever see them. My eating-disordered, black-and-white thought process convinced me that a grade of B meant I had failed. For me, it was all or nothing, and I had superhuman expectations of myself. When I started the Alliance, I truly believed that in a year, all by myself, I would be able to create a national presence for my organization, I'd have public service announcements on television, and there would be branches throughout the country. Boy, was I ever wrong! I simply wasn't being realistic. I was still thinking in black-and-white and having unreasonable expectations of myself.

Whereas previously any kind of failure would have immediately thrown me into a bottom-drawer frame of mind, I can now see that maybe I was hoping for top-drawer, but I can be okay with knowing that today is going to be a second- or third-drawer kind of day.

Underneath it all, I'm still a perfectionist. But now, when I realize that something isn't going to turn out as perfectly as I'd intended or envisioned it, I'm able to take a step back and see which parts are good and which parts are not so good, and overall, I am able to see that I really did the best I could. Whereas previously any kind of failure would have immediately thrown me into a bottom-drawer frame of mind, I can now see that maybe I was hoping for top-drawer, but I can be okay with knowing that today is going to be a second- or third-drawer kind of day. I've learned to take a look at the all, take a look at the nothing and be satisfied with something in between.

But, I am not perfect—far from it, actually. At my core, I'm still a perfectionist, which means that I still have those days (although I am so grateful that they are now much fewer and farther between) when one negative event or comment will send me directly to that bottom drawer without passing Go (and no, I do not get to collect $200). Now, however, when that happens, I know I have to take a deep breath, regroup and keep putting one foot in front of the other, even if I'm taking only baby steps. I might also ask one of my floaties for a hug, just because.

To Build an Army, You Will Need to Recruit Some Soldiers

I couldn't have learned to tame my perfectionism, to get a better perspective on myself, to increase the volume of my positive voice or to see how my eating disorder was actually ruling my life—in other words, I wouldn't have been able to get healthy—without the help and support of my therapist, my nutritionist, my treatment team, my friends and family, and my commitment. At first it was difficult for me to recruit that help, because for a long time I had felt as if I were all alone, marching against a vast enemy army. Even though they were relatives and friends, I felt as if they were all marching straight at me and I was trying to buck the tide, so to speak. What I needed to realize was that they weren't there to defeat me but to walk beside me toward a shared destination— my recovery. I actually had to visualize picking them up and moving them from in front of me to my side. That way, I could view their help as supportive rather than threatening.

The first step on my journey to recovery was determining that I could not live with my eating disorder anymore; it was no longer working for me and it was very slowly making who I was disappear. In fact, it actually got to a point when it became harder to live with my eating disorder than it was to live without it.

*It actually got to a point when it became
harder to live with my eating disorder
than it was to live without it.*

The second step, which was the key to implementing the first, was realizing that I wasn't superhuman. I couldn't do it all by myself. I needed to get help. I needed to seek guidance from people who would be able to direct me when I wasn't yet able to see the road ahead. My treatment team served as my navigation system until I was able to read the map on my own.

*My treatment team served as my
navigation system until I was able
to read the map on my own.*

My progression, although slow, probably wasn't so different from that of many others out there. It went something like this:

1. At first people try to help you, but you're not ready to accept what they have to tell you. Their help just goes in one ear and out the other. You are in denial of the problem.
2. You are ready to choose recovery and to get healthy. You take out your white crayon and go to your therapist/nutritionist/health-care provider, but

even though you're willing to listen, you're not *ready* to listen. You leave the professional's office clutching only your black crayon.

3. You get to the point where you're ready to listen, but you feel that you just *can't* do what you need to do.

4. Finally, you get to the point where you choose to make just one change. It scares you, but you do it. You took a chance, and you need to praise yourself for the risk you have taken.

5. Over time you listen more and apply what you learn more and more consistently. It's not going to be perfect, but you are willing to keep taking that next step. This will be easier at some times than others. There will be times when you feel you are going backward, but remember, even when you feel that way you are still moving forward because you are learning about yourself and your recovery.

6. At some point you feel as if you're stuck with one foot in recovery and the other in your eating disorder. This is when you need to dig in, hold on tight and do whatever it takes to put your weight on the foot that's moving you forward.

7. Eventually you realize that making healthy choices has become more second nature, and you are taking care of yourself, facing forward and continuously putting one foot in front of the other.

8. You are sitting in a room telling others your story, and you realize that your life no longer revolves around your eating disorder. You can honestly say that you are *recovered*.

Along the path, you have to constantly remind yourself that you are still human. Remember that recovery and life are not going to be perfect. When these potentially triggering people, places and things emerge, reach out for support, make yourself accountable and use the plethora of tools you have acquired throughout your journey.

Remember that recovery and life are not going to be perfect. When these potentially triggering people, places and things emerge, reach out for support.

Also, keep reminding yourself of all the people you have in your support network—not only your therapist and nutritionist but also your family, your friends, the people who may be in your support group. Basically, these are the people you know you can always call upon at any hour of the day or night. I suggest that you take the time to actually write their names down so that you can look at this list when you're feeling stuck or overwhelmed or in need, and remind yourself that you are not alone in this.

Your Recovery Affects Others, Too

I've already said that I could never have recovered without a great deal of help and support from many people, but I also noticed—and I believe you will, too—that as I was getting better, my recovery was affecting the way other people were acting and reacting to me.

Very often the significant people in our lives take on particular roles—a parent or a partner may be the caregiver; a sibling or a friend may be a cheerleader; someone in your life may be a protector, an enabler or a partner in your eating disorder behaviors. As you become stronger and begin to change, these people may find that their particular role has been written out of the script. When that happens, these significant people may feel a bit lost and perhaps even marginalized. Some of them—such as those who have shared in your eating disorder—may no longer have a place in your life at all unless they can also get help for themselves and make their own commitment to health. Sometimes people whom you may have considered floaties when your were in the midst of your eating disorder—perhaps because they were enabling your destructive behaviors—can actually turn out to be sinkies. If you feel uneasy when you're with someone, if you feel weighted down and unable to fly, you really need to weigh the pros and cons of that relationship and, if necessary, let it go.

Most people, however, want you to get better, but when you do they don't know how to adapt to the change. The people who are important in your life and who will be your support system are going through a process of change just as you are, which is why I am such a huge fan of family therapy and friends/family support groups. They need support as much as you do, even if they may not be aware of that need and may even resist getting help, at least at first. If someone is resistant, you really have to let him know that *you need* him to get support—for himself as well as for you. By getting support for themselves, your friends and family demonstrate their investment in you and learn to perform their supporting role even better so that they don't get written out of the script completely.

Keep Track of Your Mile Markers So You'll Know When You've Arrived

Each day there will be little moments that remind you how far you've come on your road to recovery. Those are your mile markers. You won't necessarily hear trumpets blaring and angels singing while holding up a banner that says, "Congratulations! You have passed another milestone in your recovery," but as you keep track of those mile markers, one day you'll realize that your eating disorder is no longer a part of your life.

Declare an Eating-Disorder-Free Zone

When you're in the process of recovering, it's vitally important that your entire life does not revolve only around your recovery. If it did, you would simply be recreating what it was like when your life revolved around your eating disorder. You are more than your eating disorder and more than your recovery.

Go out with friends who are not intimately involved with your recovery. Go to a movie or the mall. Make plans to go to the zoo, a butterfly garden, an arts-and-crafts class or even a play. Talk about anything *except* your recovery and your eating disorder. If you live with your parents, a roommate or a spouse/significant other, make sure to schedule some time out that has nothing to do with your treatment or recovery process. Doing this will reinforce your understanding that you are not your eating disorder. And it is also a wonderful way to discover what it is you like and what you have to share with those around you. It is only then that your true identity is able to emerge.

You are not your eating disorder.

It's also equally important for your family members to have a life that does not revolve entirely around your recovery. They need their own space in order to maintain their mental and emotional health so they can be present for you when you need them.

Each day there will be little moments that remind you how far you've come on your road to recovery. As you keep track of those mile markers, one day you'll realize that your eating disorder is no longer a part of your life.

Maybe you'll notice that you can sit on the couch for two hours watching TV and doing nothing else, that you're looking forward to sharing a meal with friends, that the thought of eating in a restaurant no longer makes you anxious, that you can color outside the lines in a coloring book or that you think of food as fuel (and maybe even pleasure) rather than as an enemy. The world is no longer purely black-and-white. Colors and shades of color (including gray) have now appeared and are actually pleasurable!

You're not going to be an entirely different person; you'll be who you are, but a healthier version of you.

You'll become aware that your eating disorder is no longer taking center stage in your mind, your soul, your spirit. It's no longer calling the shots. And when you do, you'll know that you're recovered.

Keep Track of Your Progress

To help you keep track of the distance you've traveled, buy yourself a little notebook and decorate it with images of things that make you feel good, which could be anything from soaring birds to a bright sun to your beloved pet. Use this as a kind of bankbook in which you record all the "deposits" you've made in your recovery bank. After a while you'll see that they begin to add up to quite a significant little nest egg. And you'll find that each deposit builds on the previous ones—like interest accrued—as one step leads to the next.

You're not going to be an entirely different person; you'll be who you are, but a healthier version of you. And you won't return to the place where you were before your eating disorder. If you did that, you'd still allow all those old triggers to dictate your thoughts and behavior. But now you have the knowledge and the tools that will allow you to respond differently—in a way that takes you to a better place of your own choosing.

Chapter Six

BEWARE OF FAKE SECURITY BLANKETS

No person is your friend who demands your silence,

or denies your right to grow.

—ALICE WALKER

I WAS WELL INTO MY RECOVERY and had moved back home to start the Alliance when one afternoon I went clothes shopping with my mother. She had bought a dress for a special occasion and was looking for an undergarment to smooth her lumps and bumps under that dress. What she bought was shapewear, a one-piece, elasticized item that marketed itself as every woman's secret weapon. It promised to slim and flatter your body in whatever you were wearing and seemed to make every figure flaw disappear.

I was in awe. I have to say that I've never met a person with an eating disorder who didn't have some kind of difficulty with or distortion of his/her body image. After all, the way so many of us chose to seek some sense of (false) control over our life was to try to take control of our body. The part of my body I was always most uncomfortable with is my midsection, so when I saw what that shapewear did for my mother, I had to buy a piece for myself, and when

I put it on, I immediately felt held in and controlled. (*Control*—wow, there's that word again.)

Initially, I told myself that it would be only for special occasions, to wear under a dress. Before long, however, I was acquiring more and more pieces of shapewear and wearing them every day, even under my jeans and T-shirts, until it got to the point where I, quite literally, would not leave the house without what I believed to be my magical undergarment. Yes, I was by then doing a much better job of taking care of myself, "doing the next right thing," and nourishing myself, but I hadn't undergone a personality transplant. My obsessive tendencies had instead found yet another outlet for expression. My shapewear made me feel secure and hidden—very much the way my eating disorder had made me feel for so long.

My shapewear made me feel secure and hidden—very much the way my eating disorder had made me feel for so long.

Over the years of trying out and wearing different styles and brands of shapewear, I settled on a version comprising a spaghetti-strap tank top with an extra-thick, extra-wide elastic waistband. (Sounds comfortable, right?) When I first went clothes shopping with my girlfriends while encased in my trusty shapewear, they asked why I was wearing such an archaic contraption. I made excuses about why I had to wear it, and over time they just stopped asking. Even my little cousin wanted to know why I wore that silly-looking bra, and I told her it was a special kind that big girls wore.

Then I started dating my husband, Max. The first time he put a hand on my waist and felt my shapewear (because you could definitely feel it, even see it, through my clothing), I think I might have told him I was wearing it to support my bad back. Amazing how easily we return to lying to keep our addictions alive! Soon Max started to call it my "body armor." He had already figured out, even though I hadn't yet, that I was using the thick and protective shapewear as a way to separate myself from the world and to make sure no one got too close to me. When I finally realized the significance of what I'd been doing, it came as a shock to me. Here I was working with other people who were overcoming eating disorders, and at the same time I was wearing my body armor to shield myself from the world. I, Johanna, had actually become addicted to my underwear! I vowed that, with the help of my therapist and Max, I would one day not have to wear my armor anymore.

I, Johanna, had actually become
addicted to my underwear!

Then, one night, there was a cold snap in South Florida—meaning that it might have gone all the way down to forty-five degrees. Max's sister, to whom I'd grown close and who knew all about my shapewear addiction, had a fireplace in her home. She called and told me that it was time to break it off with my underwear. She was going to build a fire and she wanted me to come over with all my shapewear so that we could burn it up! After many sessions with my therapist and many hours of working through why I'd been hiding behind this shield of armor, I was ready. Just like the first time I went to my nutritionist's office, metaphorically clutching my white crayon, I was willing to give up the body armor, but I was also very apprehensive.

Max and I went over to my sister-in-law's house, and I took every piece of shapewear I had (by that time I had quite a collection). I said my goodbyes and threw the first piece into the fire. What none of us had considered, however, was that the spandex, or whatever the stuff was made of, would liquefy in the heat! The first piece began to melt like the Wicked Witch of the West in *The Wizard of Oz*. As we watched in shock and amazement, it slowly disappeared. That actually felt very therapeutic and liberating. I felt as if I had been able to remove a significant chunk of one of the bricks I'd been carrying in my backpack of life. So I threw in a second piece and then a third. The fire suddenly flared up and consumed a dried wreath that was hanging above the mantelpiece. And here I had thought my eating disorder was stubborn! That shapewear was not going down without a fight! We started stomping on the wreath and quickly extinguished the fire.

My body armor was relentless and it almost took me down, but I am pleased to report that in the end, I was victorious….and we all survived!

That should have been enough to let me know it was time to quit, but I was on a roll and I wanted to continue. I kept throwing more and more pieces into the fire until it really started to smell a little funny and all three of us started to feel a bit sick. What came next, I am sure you can guess. By the end of the evening we were so sick that we all wound up in the emergency room with toxic fume inhalation poisoning. My body armor was relentless and it almost took me down, but I am pleased to report that in the end, I was victorious…and we all survived!

Reaffirm Your Connection with an Old Friend

Getting comfortable with your body when you're recovering from an eating disorder is very similar to getting reacquainted with that old friend we talked about—the one you haven't seen for a long time. You need a bit of time to get comfortable again with the skin you're in, and it's not going to happen overnight.

One technique that helped me a lot was to use positive affirmations. The first time my therapist introduced me to the concept of affirmations—saying a positive phrase to yourself until you come to believe it—I have to admit that I laughed out loud. I really thought they were silly, hokey and would never work for me. I could never imagine myself standing in front of a mirror and trying to convince myself to believe the words I was saying. But after months of persuasion I finally decided to try it, if only to appease her, even though I was still certain the exercise wouldn't do anything for me.

The first affirmation my therapist and I came up with together consisted of just two little words that had huge meaning. Although very simple, they were among the most difficult words for me to say to myself. My affirmation was "I deserve." For the longest time I hadn't believed those two words could ever apply to me. I wrote them in my journal, put them up on my mirror, printed them on index cards I kept next to my bed. Everywhere I turned, there was my affirmation staring back at me. I really needed all those reminders to say them to myself. At first I couldn't even say them out loud and had to wholeheartedly commit to the theory that I could fake it till I made it. I didn't always believe what I was telling myself, but if I kept on saying it *as if* I believed it, I thought I might eventually internalize those thoughts. And to my amazement, it worked. The more I said those words to myself, the more I started to believe them. I can now say that I fully appreciate the power of affirmations to reframe one's thought process. What's important, however, is that you have conviction in your voice. There's no room here for what I call conditional punctuation. Saying "I'm special?" or "I deserve?"

with that question mark at the end isn't going to convince you. If you hear that uncertainty creeping into your voice, you need to replace the question mark with a definitive exclamation point! And make sure to say it out loud. Imagine that there is a person standing on the other side of the room, and make sure he or she can hear it, too!

My affirmation was "I deserve." I wrote those words in my journal, put them up on my mirror, printed them on index cards I kept next to my bed. The more I said those words to myself, the more I started to believe them.

Affirmations are very personal, so the ones that worked for me may not resonate for you, but here are a few you might like. Of course, you should feel free to make up your own or seek out one of the many books available that focus on affirmations.

- I will treat my body with love and respect.
- I am okay with being okay.
- I am special.
- I deserve to be happy.
- I respect and cherish my body and all its amazing functions.
- I treat myself with the respect I deserve.
- I accept and embrace myself.
- Finding out who I am doesn't have to be hard.
- I am really grateful for who I am and everything I have accomplished.
- I cannot be everything to everybody. I cannot expect anyone to be everything to me.
- I believe in myself and respect myself.

And finally, here's one you should always remember: *I am more than my weight and appearance. I am me and that is just fabulous.*

Sometimes a Security Blanket Might Not Be a Blanket at All

When I was a little girl, I had a baby blanket. It was made of white crocheted yarn and was adorned with little pink roses. I took it everywhere, and as long as it was with me I felt protected and safe. My mom had even told me that as long as I had the blanket with me, I would be okay. I had it with me when I played, when I slept, when I was with family—basically all the time. Even during those nights when I was afraid of the dark, my blanket always made me feel safer. As I got older and it became uncool to carry a blanket around, it started to stay home while I went to school or out to play. Then after a while the blanket, although it had great sentimental value, did not have the same comforting powers anymore. I saw it for what it was—a little crocheted square of yarn that was by now worn and fraying at the seams. I didn't want to throw it away because of the significance it had held for me, so I folded it up and put it away underneath some boxes on a closet shelf. At some point, my security blanket had played a truly positive role in my life; in fact, I now see it as my very first floatie.

I am more than my weight and appearance.
I am me and that is just fabulous.

So what's the difference between my positive security blanket and my body armor? Answer: the fact that my body armor was never truly a floatie! Like my eating disorder, the shapewear was an imposter, a sinkie disguising itself as a floatie. While it's okay to keep a positive security blanket you no longer need stashed away on the shelf, where you know you can take it out from time to time, say thank you for what it did in the past and put it away again, you can't hold on to a fake and unsafe security blanket. You need to get rid of it once and for all (even if, like my shapewear, it fights you every inch of the way), because if you don't do that, it might sink you.

In the grand scheme of things, it now seems amazing that my eating disorder originally presented itself like my baby blanket. At a time when I needed it the most, my eating disorder made me feel safe, in control and protected from life, just as my baby blanket had protected me from the dark. But as I sank further into my disease and continued to wrap that "security blanket" around me, what had once been comfort actually turned into suffocation. I had been deceived; my eating disorder was an imposter—a fake security blanket.

My eating disorder was an imposter—
a fake security blanket.

You just need to be hyperaware. When a situation, or a person, for that matter, you have thought of as supportive is actually holding you back or pulling you down, you need to let it go. There's no definitive way for me to tell you which is which. Fake security blankets are as individual as the paths we took to develop our eating disorder and the paths we take to recovery. All I can say is that when you get an uneasy feeling in your gut, you need to stop and examine that feeling. Figure out where it's coming from and why. Your brain may play tricks on you, but your gut doesn't lie.

The Danger of Trading One Addiction for Another

As I said, when I committed myself to recovery and even after I was no longer engaging in destructive eating behaviors, I was still Johanna. I hadn't traded in my personality for a different model; I hadn't upgraded to version 2.0. So I was still one of those people who tend to think in black-and-white. I still needed to be vigilant about falling into addictive, obsessive behaviors. And initially, that was exactly what I did with my body armor.

Again, I'm not unique. I remember one member of our support group, named Leah, who began battling anorexia at the age of twenty-four and struggled for fourteen years before she asked for help. She had gone into an inpatient program and absorbed everything she could to help her get better. But even though she said she was willing to recover, there were still many important aspects of her struggle that she was not willing to face or work through. She did what she was supposed to do throughout her inpatient treatment, and when she left she really believed she was finally on a healthy path.

Now that her eating disorder was no longer occupying her thoughts every moment of every day, she determined to move to the next level in her career as a real estate broker. She had worked as a receptionist in a real estate office before she entered treatment and had always wanted to become a broker. Through networking, doing research on the top real estate companies in her area and making a lot of phone calls, she found what she considered an ideal job with a top-rated company. She worked on her résumé, bought a new suit and went for the interview. After a pretty intense interview process, she found out that she had gotten the job. Now she was determined to become the perfect employee and the best worker her company ever had. (Is this sounding familiar?) She worked longer and harder than anyone else in her office. She began to eat, breathe and live her job. She stopped making dates with her friends on weekdays so that she could stay in the office later. And she went into the office on weekends, even though no one had asked her or expected her to do so. She was constantly being praised as a model employee, and the recognition made her feel good. Leah's job had become her life. It became her new version of all or nothing, black or white. It was entitling her to escape from living her life to the fullest in the same way her eating disorder had done.

Then came the economic meltdown and downsizing of 2008, and despite her stellar job performance, her firm went out of business and she lost her job. And what happened then? She went right back to her disordered eating behaviors.

Like me with my shapewear, Leah had become addicted to her job. Instead of sublimating everything else in her life to her eating disorder, she'd transferred her identity and black-and-white thinking and behavior to her job. She had traded in her eating disorder for this "perfect" job. She'd invested everything in a fake security blanket. So, when she lost her job, she had nothing to fall back on but her eating disorder. She felt as if she had fallen from top-drawer to bottom-drawer in no time at all.

I'm happy to say that Leah went back into treatment and got back on Recovery Road. She now has a new job and makes sure to keep herself accountable to her therapist to be certain that she doesn't get sucked back into the same self-sabotaging behavior.

Basically, I am very grateful that I was lucky enough—with the help of all my floaties—to have become aware of what I was doing before my shapewear had a chance to snap back and drag me back down an even unhealthier path.

Never Put All Your Marbles in One Jar

The lesson to be learned here is that "all or nothing" is never a healthy choice. We need to be careful that we are not just substituting another unhealthy behavior for our eating disorder. Imagine for a moment that you are looking at a jar and some marbles. What words would you use to describe that jar? Here are a few that come to my mind: *clear, glass* and *breakable*. Now imagine putting all the marbles in that jar. The problem with doing that is that if the jar breaks (which is a possibility because it is made out of glass) or if the top isn't screwed on and it tips over, your marbles will roll all over the place and some of them may even land in a hard-to-reach place, like under the couch, from where they will be hard to retrieve.

Do not put all your "marbles" of recovery into one jar.

When you start the recovery process, it is very important that you do not put all your "marbles" of recovery into one jar, because you don't want to risk losing everything you've been working so hard to build up. If Leah had worked to pursue more of her interests outside of her job, she wouldn't have felt so lost when her one safety net—her job—was taken away from her. That's one of the main reasons why it's so important to think about the things you like, the things that support you and the things that make you smile, and write them down. After a while, you may be surprised to realize how many facets there really are to you and your life. You may be delighted to discover that like an uncut diamond, your rough, opaque exterior has been hiding your innate sparkle and depth.

Where Do You Put Your Marbles?

To help you truly see your unique diversity, go out and invest in a few glass jars and bags of marbles. It's worth it because what you're really doing is investing in yourself.

Now, label your jars: support, work, fun, hobbies, successes, friends—whatever you think reflects something that makes you you. Then, think of all the things that fill up each of those aspects of your life. If you need help, take out and review the lists you've been making. You can even ask a friend or family member to remind you of something they love, appreciate or admire about you. For each trait, activity, person or thing you can think of that contributes to one of those categories, put a marble in the appropriate jar.

Then, each time you do something to support yourself, achieve a success, take a risk or do something that brings you pleasure, put a marble in the jar where it belongs. All those marbles represent your personal floaties, the people and things that have supported you on your journey. Before long, you'll see how full your jars—and your life—have become.

Another Way of Looking at It: Diversification of Assets

Experts in the financial world generally agree that spreading your assets among varied kinds of investments is the single most important key to developing a healthy portfolio. By doing that, you are minimizing potential losses. In fact, the gains in your other investments may offset any losses you incur. Sounds a lot like everyday life and the recovery process, right? A financial advisor will tell you to diversify with three basic tools: liquid assets like money market funds or CDs, bonds and stocks. The liquid investments are considered short-term and low risk, bonds are generally longer term and moderate risk, and stocks are most likely to provide you with the greatest return but are also the highest risk. Just as we have to diversify our financial investments, it is extremely important to diversify our investments in the recovery process and not put all our marbles in one jar.

So How Do You Diversify Your Recovery Funds?

Applying the theory of diversifying assets to your recovery process can prove to be a great investment and yield very high returns for your recovery. If you could apply the theories of the financial world to your journey, what would your portfolio look like?

Take out a sheet of paper and divide it into three sections. At the top of each section write: Short-Term Liquid Investments, Bonds/Long-Term Investments and Stocks/High-Risk Investments. Your short-term liquid investments are the things you do on a daily basis to take care of yourself. Your long-term investments are your long-term goals. Your high-risk investments are those risky choices that can potentially earn you tremendous returns. Now, take a moment to think about what you would put under each of these headings and write them down. Here's an example of what your "portfolio" might look like:

Short-Term Liquid Investments

- Doing the next right thing toward my recovery
- Going to my therapist, nutritionist, physician, family therapy, support group, etc.
- Saying affirmations

Bonds/Long-Term Investments

- Going back to school/work
- Creating and maintaining interpersonal networks
- Being okay with the okay
- Focusing on being happy and healthy
- Living each day and thriving

Stocks/High-Risk Investments

- Picking up the phone and making "that" call when I really need to talk
- Applying for a job
- Making new friends
- Taking food risks
- Using my voice

Let Go of the Old to Grab Hold of the New You

We tend to hang on to behaviors that represent or negatively replace our eating disorder. I did it with my body armor, Leah did it with her job, and you may be doing it with your own fake security blanket. If so, once again, I can't emphasize enough how important it is to let go of them, because if your life is filled up with negative, self-limiting thoughts and behaviors, there won't be any room to let the new, positive stuff in. Don't put all your marbles (or your efforts) in one jar. Diversify the many assets you already have and will be acquiring, and use each one of them to build upon the next. Eventually you'll find that you're richer than you had ever dreamed you could be.

When I first met Jamie, I was amazed by the similarity of our stories. Although we grew up in different places and came from different backgrounds, her story could have been mine. It made me realize that no matter what your struggle is, you are never alone. There are people out there who are experiencing and feeling the same things as you are. To me that just reinforces my belief in the importance of using your voice and reaching out. Her honesty and bravery inspire me, the women in my support group and all those with whom she works on a daily basis. She is living proof that recovery is possible and worth it.

If you had asked me three years ago whether I believed I would ever be able to share my story of recovery, my response most likely would have been a hopeless no. For me, the idea of living without an eating disorder, especially *my* eating disorder, was incomprehensible. For nearly eleven years my eating disorder was my friend, my safety net, my armor and my identity. By starving, purging and exercising away the self-hatred, worries and struggles that lay within my heart and mind, I thought I was opening myself up to loving others more fully. I truly believed that with an eating disorder, I could do anything and everything. Reflecting back upon those years, I now realize that the honeymoon period with my eating disorder ended soon after my struggle began. Over time, I have come to understand that I was engaging in a deceitful and unforgiving relationship with myself. I was a prisoner in my own skin. This is my story....

When I was in sixth grade, my life changed forever with one comment from my dance teacher, whom I truly adored and admired. Yes, I probably had the genetic predisposition to developing an eating disorder, but the environment in which I found my passion was not the most conducive to preventing its onset. It all began when I was not accepted at a summer dance camp. I was accepted at four others but could not understand why I had been denied admission to that one in particular. When I discussed my summer camp options with my dance teacher, she stated that I was going to have a tough time in the years to come because I would continuously battle with my body weight, size and shape. According to her, since my father was overweight, I was destined to be overweight as well, and I would never be as successful as dancers who had the "ideal dancer's body."

For nearly eleven years my eating disorder was my friend, my safety net, my armor and my identity.

I wanted my dance teacher to see me in a different light. I wanted her to see me as the perfect dancer I desired to be. So, for nearly five years, from seventh through twelfth grades, I followed the same daily routine as I dressed for ballet class: use the restroom (to purge if necessary), tape blisters, carefully put on seamed pink tights and a black leotard, pull my hair tightly and perfectly into a bun, sit and slip on pointe shoes, swallow two extra-strength painkillers and snap on a tummy belt. *Plié, tendu, balancé, échappé, fouetté, grand jeté, pas de chat, penché, pirouette, rond de jambe en l'air* and *saut de basque* were just a few of the many French words and phrases that became my second language. The dance studio became my second home. Every part of my being loved dancing because it was my way of expressing myself and releasing any emotion that occupied my mind. Others recognized my talent and my passion, and I embraced the identity of a dancer and a person with an eating disorder. For me the two were inseparable.

....

I was a prisoner in my own skin.

....

As part of this identity, I was not allowed to make a mistake, experience physical pain or expose my self-hatred. I was supposed to be perfect. Fighting against hunger and denying myself food were expressions of my effort to become perfect. I was striving to live up to the expectations I had of myself—to be the perfect dancer, the perfect student, the perfect daughter, the perfect sister and the perfect friend.

....

I was striving to live up to the expectations I had of myself—to be the perfect dancer, the perfect student, the perfect daughter, the perfect sister and the perfect friend.

....

Even though I had many friends and a family who clearly thought I was lovable, I believed that being thin would make me more perfect and, therefore, more lovable. The thinner I was, the more love I could and would receive—or so I thought.

My eating disorder voice told me that being thin was the key to being loved, but in my journey to recovery I came to realize that this was not true. In reality, it was a lie my eating disorder loved to tell me.

When I entered college I began to get frustrated with my struggle. Unfortunately, my belief that if I quit dancing my eating disorder would go away also turned out to be untrue. Rather, when I stopped dancing, I became involved in NCAA Division I rowing. I signed up for twenty-plus hours of training, and my eating disorder fully supported that commitment. Before I knew it, I was exercising up to four hours per day, counting every calorie that entered my mouth and isolating myself from my closest friends in an effort to hide what I knew was not normal behavior. Once again I was striving for perfection. I wanted to be the fastest, strongest and leanest person on my team. We practiced indoors using rowing machines, and for me, each practice was a fight for my seat in the top boat—until I collapsed after a practice race and needed medical attention.

··

I believed that being thin would make me more perfect and, therefore, more lovable. The thinner I was, the more love I could and would receive—or so I thought.

··

Dehydration was the diagnosis, but fluids were not the only thing I received from this event. I was forced to enter therapy by the athletic department and my coach and was told that I must see a physician weekly. I would have to be cleared by a psychologist and a physician before I could return to regular practices with the team. While I was not yet ready to begin recovery, I had to face my eating disorder and began to entertain the idea of seeking help.

Over the years, my eating disorder placed me in a wrist cast from falling while running, in a walking cast from a stress fracture due to overexercise, on crutches from a sprained ankle and finally in therapy to address my eating disorder; in a doctor's office for medical clearance, checkups and blood work; and in the hospital to replace fluids that I'd lost through restricting and purging. Most important to me, however, was the emotional pain that my family and closest friends had endured as a result of my eating disorder. At that point, I did not want to find out where or what the next stop on the path of self-destruction might be.

My journey to recovery has not been easy or smooth, but it has been memorable. It took many hours of therapy, nutrition counseling, journaling and attending support groups, plus a strong willingness to choose recovery with each new day. There were many times when I wanted to throw in the towel and give up because the fight seemed too much for me to handle. Fortunately, my support system and treatment team were there to help me at every wrong turn and obstacle I encountered.

> I now live my life free from the grips of an eating disorder. I wake up and go through my day without having to weigh myself or my worth. I eat without having to know how many calories are in the food.

I now live my life free from the grips of an eating disorder. I wake up and go through my day without having to weigh myself or my worth. I eat without having to know how many calories are in the food. I shop for clothing and walk out with full shopping bags! Admittedly, there are still days when I find myself being critical of my body weight, size and/or shape, but I no longer allow those negative thoughts to determine my mood or how I will interact with others. Rather, I let them pass and do not allow them to ruin my day.

Each day I make the choice to continue walking the path toward being recovered. I have learned that this path is as much about discovery as it

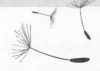

is about recovery. Each new day I am blessed to experience is another day I choose to put my best foot forward and work to maintain my recovery. Never would I have thought I would be saying this, but I offer you these words: recovery is possible and worth it!

<hr>

> My wish for those of you who are struggling is that you find the courage to face the demon that is your eating disorder. My wish for those of you who are on the journey to recovery is that you continue to find the courage to keep putting one foot in front of the other.

<hr>

My wish for those of you who are struggling is that you find the courage to face the demon that is your eating disorder. My wish for those of you who are on the journey to recovery is that you continue to find the courage to keep putting one foot in front of the other. We are all blessed with one life, and what I now know is that life is *so* much better free from the grips of an eating disorder.

Chapter Seven

GETTING TO THE HEART
OF THE ARTICHOKE

I don't look to jump over seven-foot bars;
I look around for one-foot bars that I can step over.
— WARREN BUFFETT

PEOPLE OFTEN COMPARE THE THERAPEUTIC process to peeling back the layers of an onion. You start with the exterior paperlike skin and work your way through the layers to get to the center. It seems to make a lot of sense, but realistically, if you have ever peeled an onion, you know that it can make you cry and the skin can be very sticky. And, beyond that, once you've peeled away all the layers, there's nothing left!

So, what I'd like you to do is to visualize an artichoke instead of an onion. If you've ever eaten an artichoke, you know that it can be a lot of work. One by one you pull off those thick, prickly outer leaves, scrape off the little bit of sweet meat at the base and keep going until you get to the soft, tender heart. In my mind, the recovery process is more like eating an artichoke than peeling an onion. Steady as you go, and you will make it to the heart or, shall we say, your goal.

The recovery process is like eating an artichoke.
Steady as you go, and you will make it to the heart.

Are You Willing?

The first question my therapist asked me all those years ago was "Are you willing?" I still remember as if it were yesterday how that question made me feel. It was overwhelming and very scary. After taking a few minutes to think about it, I could honestly answer that although I wasn't ready to commit fully to the recovery process, yes, I was willing to consider it. Now, whenever a new member joins our support group, I, too, ask that question. The only requirement I have of anyone is that he or she be willing to face the prospect of recovery. But not too long ago one new member, whom I'll call Diana, told me that after I'd posed that question, she'd gone to her therapist and said, "Maybe I shouldn't go back to group." When I asked what about the question had been so overwhelming for her, she said that she was willing to *think* about getting better but she wasn't yet willing to give up her eating disorder entirely, because life would be too hard and too scary without it.

I'm not asking you to walk through the door,
slam it behind you, lock the dead bolt and be done
with your eating disorder. All I ask of anyone is that
you be willing to crack open the door and peek out.

Diana was still caught up in her black-and-white thinking, and she immediately assumed there was no way to recover except to give it all up right away and be done with it. But that wasn't what I was asking. In fact, it was just the opposite. I'm not asking you to walk through the door, slam it behind you, lock the dead bolt and be done with your eating disorder. All I ask of anyone is that you be willing to crack open the door and peek out. What you see when you take that peek might be a little scary, if only because it is still the unknown. Therefore, you *need* to take it slow. Recovery is not a sprint to the finish line. There are no deadlines and no time clocks. Willingness is not a black-or-white issue. It's what you need to start the process and to keep you going when you need to face an issue that may be really tough to look at. When I first began leading support groups, I used to ask new members to imagine their lives without an eating disorder. But I soon realized even that was asking too much. Many, if not most, of us don't even know who we would be without our eating disorder. For most people — myself included — our eating disorder is so central to our lives that, initially, we believe that without it we'd have to completely reinvent ourselves. We'd have to become totally different people, and we'd be left with no coping skills at all.

Recovery is not a sprint to the finish line.
There are no deadlines and no time clocks.

If your eating disorder is your one way of coping with the world, you assume that without it you'll feel totally naked, stripped of your armor. And, quite naturally, you don't even want to think about how that would feel. But that's not how it is; actually, it's quite the opposite.

Try Out New and Better Tools

The beauty of recovery is that you're never without coping tools. What you do is find new, healthier ways to cope. You pick up one tool at a time and try it out. Some will feel comfortable. You'll be able to use them, and you'll put them in your toolbox to use when you need them. Others won't feel comfortable at all. They won't work for you, and you'll discard them. There's no shame in that. It's all about keeping what works, discarding what doesn't and not putting all your marbles in one jar. Recovery is about knowing that you have options. Having many tools gives you many options.

Start with the Outer Leaves

So, what has all this got to do with eating an artichoke? (Yes, we are back to the artichoke...I hadn't forgotten.) Well, as I've said, it can take some work, and you've got to be willing to persevere through the prickly parts in order to get to the heart. In fact, those prickly outer leaves do for the artichoke exactly what your eating disorder behaviors have been doing for you—covering up, hiding and protecting the fragile, vulnerable heart of the vegetable, or in your case, protecting you from having to feel anything at all. I know that in my case, I was afraid to face the world because I never felt pretty enough or smart enough or good enough at anything, and my eating disorder was something I felt I was very good at. I was good at restricting, then bingeing and purging, and at compulsive overeating. I was good at manipulating everyone and everything and keeping my secret. So, perversely, my eating disorder behaviors allowed me to feel good about myself. Isn't it amazing how we can feel so good about being so self-destructive?

Filling Your Toolbox

When you are in the process of filling your recovery toolbox, you might choose a tool that you think will be useful and then discover that it's not working for you. At that point you may be tempted to slam the lid shut and forget the whole thing. But I beg you, please don't do that. It can take some time to find the tools that will resonate for you, so please be willing to keep trying.

What I have found really helpful is to talk to people you trust and ask them what they have in their recovery toolboxes. Your toolbox is, essentially, like a football team's playbook. They have worked out a variety of plays they can use depending upon the situation. They need these options because they don't know exactly how the game is going to play out. And the same is true for your box of tools. Remember that some of these tools will be very helpful to you, while others might not work at all. You get to pick and choose.

To help you get started, here are some that proved helpful to me:

- A list of the tools I could turn to when I found myself triggered to act out—my personal playbook. Do not wait until the moment you are triggered to write the list. You will find that as you continue down your path, you will be adding to your list.
- Choosing one person in my support circle to whom I would be accountable. Make sure you have an understudy or two waiting in the wings in case that person can't be available to you.
- Asking three or four people I love and trust to write three things that are good about me in my playbook.
- Writing a letter to myself when I am doing the next right thing and feeling strong in my recovery so that I'd have it to read on a day when I feel defeated by my eating disorder and the recovery process.
- Having a special place to go, like the beach or a museum, where I feel safe and secure.
- My smile list. ☺

As you continue down your path to recovery, always be on the lookout for new tools to add to your toolbox. You can never have too many tools. Remember, you can always upgrade to a bigger toolbox!

*My eating disorder gave me carte blanche
not to have to do things that scared me:
I didn't have to feel. I didn't have to confront
anyone. Basically, it protected me from
having to deal with life, reality and the future.*

For once I felt as if I were in control (except, of course, I wasn't). Some people cover up their fears and escape from reality with alcohol or drugs. But those were not my escapes of choice, because I needed to be in control and know what was going on at all times. I could not deal with anything that hadn't been preplanned and thoroughly dissected. Even the thought that someone might want to give me a surprise party was enough to make me extremely uncomfortable. So, thinking that I was in charge of what I ate was the perfect out for me. It gave me a way to focus on the food and not very much else.

*Start to peel back and pull off the outer leaves
of the artichoke one by one. Look at a behavior
or thought or pattern, bite off what's good
about it and set aside what's left.*

My eating disorder was my "get out of jail free" card. It gave me carte blanche not to have to do things that scared me: I didn't have to feel. I didn't have to confront anyone. I didn't have to face what felt like the overwhelming responsibilities of becoming an adult. Basically, my eating disorder protected me from having to deal with life, reality and the future.

As you begin the recovery process, you start to peel back and pull off the outer leaves of the artichoke one by one. You look at a behavior or thought or pattern, bite off what's good about it (because, again, nothing is entirely black or white) and set aside what's left on your discard plate.

In my own case, as a student I always got my work done on time, and I hated it when the teacher assigned group projects. Invariably, I would get my portion of the project completed and then have to wait for the other members of my group to finish their sections. The night before the project was due to be turned in, if any of my group members had failed to complete the assignment, I would be frantically finishing up their work so that I would get a good grade. As a perfectionist, I couldn't let the imperfections of others reflect badly on me. As a result, I learned very early in life to do everything myself, because in order to be satisfied, I'd wind up having to do it all anyway. Although my work ethic and organizational skills were outstanding, I was extremely inflexible and virtually incapable of working with other people or asking for help.

When I started peeling back the layers of my "recovery artichoke," I had to learn that while it was great to be organized and dedicated, I could not do it all alone—no one can. I held on to the work ethic and let go of my rigidity about asking for help. Sometimes people affirmed my preconceptions by disappointing me, and sometimes they exceeded my expectations by coming through with flying colors. So, as you begin to do that for yourself, think about those leaves that were left on your discard plate and see what you can find that is good in them. How can you reframe what was originally unhealthy and use it to help you? Think about how you can modify those once unhealthy behaviors and feelings into new healthy ones even when doing what's healthy seems almost impossible. Remember—no feeling, characteristic or thought is all good or bad; it's simply how we choose to use it.

When you're peeling back the leaves of your own artichoke, some days you may be able to get through two or three leaves. Some days you'll be able to pick off only one. Some days you'll encounter a leaf that simply refuses to let go, no matter how hard you try to yank it off. And some days you'll pull off a leaf and find a whole new artichoke hiding underneath it—oh my! When that happens, set the new artichoke aside to deal with at some other time. You will get to it when you are good and ready. Do not take the sudden emergence of this new artichoke as an excuse to stop peeling the layers of the one you were already working on. Return to the original artichoke and move on to the next leaf.

If you try to do too much too soon, you could potentially feel overwhelmed. Some of the issues you bring up will be easier to deal with than others. But if you go about it slowly and methodically, before you know it, there will be more leaves on the discard plate than are still attached to the artichoke itself, and you'll be that much closer to the heart. Just remember, there is no right or wrong way to peel an artichoke.

You'll uncover issues you may not have
wanted to face for a very long time.
You're going to start feeling again,
the good and the bad, the happy and the sad.

This process is very similar to what we talked about in Chapter Two, when I suggested that you try to lighten your load by chipping away at the bricks in your backpack that have been weighing you down. I would never ask you to just start flinging whole bricks away, because that would be like slamming the door on your eating disorder and not looking back, or pulling every leaf off an artichoke all at one time. It's too much to ask and not really possible. You'd lose your ballast and your balance. It would be self-sabotage. But you can carefully chip away little pebbles, one brick at a time, and soon you'll find that you've done away with an entire brick, or maybe even two. Before you discard those broken bricks completely, take a moment to examine them. Might there be some positive characteristics and behaviors hiding among the rubble? Never forget that this is a process of discovery.

Getting to the Core

As you peel away more and more of the outer leaves of the artichoke you'll expose the stem, and you'll notice that all the parts are really connected to one another. The leaves are attached to the stem, which gradually widens to enclose the core—the heart of the matter.

As you proceed, you'll uncover issues you may not have wanted to face for a very long time. Like one of my friends, you may have days when all you want to do is take all those leaves you've peeled off, stick them right back on the artichoke and put it out of your sight and your mind. That's normal because you're going to start feeling again, the good and the bad, the happy and the sad. And sometimes you may not even know what you feel, because for so long you've tried to escape feeling altogether. For so long you have been numb.

An exercise that was really helpful for me when I first started to feel again was to look at a list of feeling words to help me figure out how I felt. Keep in mind, there is no right or wrong feeling. You might feel one way right now and a completely different way five minutes from now. Here is a list of feeling words you can refer to, to help you identify what you are feeling.

FEELING WORDS

Happy	Afraid	Positive
Content	Fearful	Proud
Glad	Uncomfortable	Inspired
Pleased	Terrified	Determined
Playful	Anxious	Brave
Fortunate	Worried	Optimistic
Important	Shaken	Thankful
Satisfied	Scared	Courageous
Great	Panicky	Alive
Thrilled	Nervous	Confident
Enthusiastic	Alarmed	Grateful
Terrific	Frightened	Strong
Free	Uneasy	Hopeful
Warm	Vulnerable	Committed

FEELING WORDS

Sad	Angry	Other
Depressed	Annoyed	Loved
Unhappy	Irritated	Okay
Empty	Enraged	Jealous
Disappointed	Grumpy	Responsible
Lonely	Frustrated	Caring
Down	Explosive	Confused
Hopeless	Upset	Curious
Withdrawn	Sore	Quiet
Heartbroken	Resentful	Blessed
Powerless	Disgusted	Rebellious
Hurt	Bitter	Unique
Rejected	Infuriated	Embarrassed
Despondent	Fed up	Comforted

And if you are a more visual person, and lists of words don't really do it for you, consider investing in Feelings Faces items (such as refrigerator magnets that say "How Are You Feeling Today?" and show faces with feeling words underneath).

And remember that those outer leaves of the artichoke have stickers at their tips, but there is also a sweet spot at the base. At first you may find that the thought of feeling good is even scarier than feeling bad, mainly because it's new and unfamiliar. We know very well what it's like to feel bad, which is why it actually feels safe. Feeling good, however, is still the unknown—and if it's unknown, we can't control it, so it's unsafe and scary.

*Gradually, you will find that you actually start **wanting** to feel good, and good will begin to feel safer than bad.*

I know I always believed that anytime I was feeling happy, something was going to happen to mess it up, and then I'd feel bad. I knew that once I allowed myself to feel good, feeling bad would be that much worse. Once you've reached that top drawer, the fall to the bottom feels a lot harder. So, time after time I kicked off the other shoe to be sure I knew where it would land. Gradually, however, you will find that you actually start *wanting* to feel good, and good will begin to feel safer than bad. It will no longer be unfamiliar to feel good.

So, again, as you slowly peel back the leaves of that artichoke, keep reminding yourself that you're getting to the sweet heart. That will be your reward. You'll notice that the closer you get, the less tough the leaves are. You're breaking down barriers, dismantling the wall you've built around yourself. You're opening your sweet heart and soul to the world. You can do that! You deserve to do that!

But—a word of caution: once you peel off all the leaves, there's still that hairy choke to get through. To me, that's a perfect metaphor for the fact that there is always work to be done. I know I'm recovered, but I'm certainly not perfect. To be honest, neither recovery nor being recovered will ever be perfect. I believe that's a good thing to know, because if you thought you had to be perfect, you'd probably be too intimidated to even begin the process!

Chapter Eight

LAILA, ROSIE, THE INCREDIBLE HULK
AND OTHER POWERFUL HEALTHY VOICES

Towanda, righter of wrongs, queen beyond compare.

—"EVELYN COUCH," *FRIED GREEN TOMATOES*

WHEN YOU'RE IN THE THROES of an eating disorder, that loud negative voice in your head may be all you hear. Your healthy voice may be nothing more than a sporadic whisper in the background that doesn't yet have the strength to insist on making itself heard.

"What you need to understand and truly believe is that your negative voice doesn't have any right to occupy that space in your brain, no matter how hard it tries to convince you that it is your friend and protector. It doesn't pay rent, it doesn't contribute anything positive to your fiscal or emotional bank account, it doesn't have a lease, and it's not a statutory tenant, so you can *evict it!* Then, when you've kicked it to the curb, you can put an ad in the classifieds for a new tenant—a constant, healthy voice that will be honest and loving.

What Does Your Ad Say?

Imagine that you really are writing that ad for a healthy voice. Before you can compose the ad, you will need to take a moment to think about what qualities you would want your healthy voice to possess. When I first approached this exercise, I was actually a lot more comfortable and familiar with my negative voice than I was with my healthy voice, so it posed a big challenge for me. To help me through the exercise, my therapist asked me to first put together a list of words that described my negative voice. Once I'd done that, I could use the list as a reference to figure out what characteristics I would need my healthy voice to have.

Here's what I came up with.

Negative voice:

- Controlling
- Critical
- Fearful
- Mean
- Degrading
- Hateful
- Manipulative
- Angry
- Isolating
- Sneaky
- Loud
- Lying

Once I got that out of the way, I determined what I wanted my positive voice to be.

Positive and healthy voice:

- Loving
- Nurturing
- Hopeful
- Safe
- Strong
- Patient
- Helpful
- Compassionate
- Accepting
- Courageous
- Trustworthy
- Loud
- Daring
- Stable
- Brave
- Rational
- Affectionate
- Fearless
- Loyal
- Consistent

You can do the same thing I did. Write down the characteristics of your negative voice and then counteract them with those of a positive, healthy voice. Once you've come up with the traits you most want in your positive voice, it's time to write your ad.

Mine looked something like this:

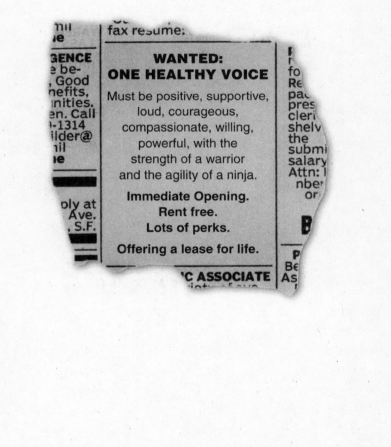

Now make up your own ad. What would it say? Feel free to use some of the characteristics listed above, and, of course, you can add some of your own. Your ad can be any length, but it must be persuasive and positive. Remember, you want to attract a really great tenant because you will hopefully be living with this healthy, positive voice for the rest of your life.

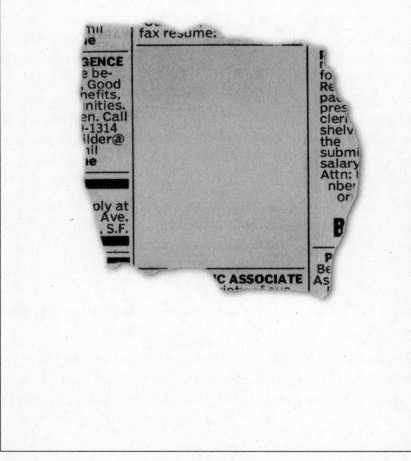

Name Your Voice

It's important to name your positive voice so that it has an identity separate from your own and can speak up for you when you're unable to use your own voice.

Whenever I ask the members of my support group what name they would choose to associate with the qualities they want in their healthy voice, I get some surprising and wonderful answers. One woman chose her grandmother's name because she said that her grandmother was the strongest, most loving and compassionate person she knew. And she said there was no other person in the world who loved her so unconditionally. That made me smile because I, too, had chosen my grandmother's name—Rosalie. (In fact, it's amazing that over the years, so many members of my groups have used their grandmothers' names for their healthy voices.) My grandmother is the epitome of strength. She has lived through wars and poverty and raised seven children in extremely difficult circumstances. She was not formally educated but she's brilliant. She is extremely loving and compassionate, yet she can also be firm and protective when necessary. When I was battling my eating disorder, I needed someone as powerful and capable as her in my corner.

Another group member said she was naming her healthy voice Rosie, after Rosie the Riveter. She imagined the famous J. Howard Miller poster in which the iconic character, wearing a red-and-white polka-dot bandana that covers her hair, has her sleeves rolled back to expose a flexed biceps. When she was looking for a positive voice, she pictured herself wearing Rosie's coveralls, holding up her fist and shouting, "We can do it. We can fight this eating disorder."

One member chose Elle Woods from the film *Legally Blonde*. What made her stand out as a great model for this woman's healthy voice was that Elle is authentic and does not really care what other people think. She defies stereotypes and stands up for what she believes in. No one has the power to stand in the way of her dreams.

Because most of my group members are women, they tend to pick female voices, but one member made me smile when she said that her voice was the Marvel Comics character the Incredible Hulk. She explained that her Hulk was wearing a T-shirt with the Nike slogan Just Do It! written across the front. What she liked about the Hulk was that he was a good guy until he was provoked. And she wanted her positive voice to be peaceful, loving and compassionate but also willing to go to the mat and fight for her when necessary.

Pick a name that's meaningful to you and come up with all the reasons your voice is both powerful and inspirational—your ultimate floatie!

What would you name your voice? Maybe you'll be inspired by "Towanda" from the film *Fried Green Tomatoes,* or by Muhammad Ali's daughter Laila, a powerful boxer in her own right. The challenge is to pick a name that's meaningful to you and come up with all the reasons your voice is both powerful and inspirational—your ultimate floatie! As you go through the recovery process, you may find that the name of the person you're picturing changes but that his or her characteristics remain very much the same. I was extremely moved when one woman whose deepest wish had always been to have a baby became pregnant after two and a half years in our group and said that she had changed the identity of her healthy voice from her grandmother's to that of her unborn child.

Change Your Focus to Change Your Mind

For many of us, the problem is that we've been ceding our power to that negative eating disorder voice for a very long time, and the more we listen to it the more powerful and scarier it becomes. So what I'm asking you to do is change your focus and listen to your healthy voice instead. By doing that, you'll be giving your healthy voice the power.

Have you ever been in a group of people where one person's voice was so loud that it seemed to drown out everyone else's conversations? Even though you might not have wanted to, it was probably difficult *not* to listen to that loud-mouth shouting in the corner. But if you turned your back on the overpowering voice and really concentrated on what the person on your other side was saying, you could stop listening to the loud voice and tune in to what you really wanted to hear.

That's all I'm asking you to do. Instead of listening to that negative voice saying, "You're not good enough" or "You can't do this" or "You don't deserve this, blah blah blah," turn your back on it and tune into your healthy voice saying, "You can do this. You deserve it. You are good enough."

Sometimes It's Hard to Do It Alone

Sometimes, when you're trying to cope with the toxicity of what your eating disorder is doing to your body and your spirit, you just don't have the strength to fight a one-person battle. You may think you're all alone, that no one understands what you're going through and that you're going to be the only person ever who isn't able to recover. But then you hear that positive voice in your head, and you know you really are strong, deserving and capable. The truth is that walking the road to recovery isn't going to be easy, but it becomes a lot easier when you have that positive voice walking with you, helping you to put one foot in front of the other and keep moving forward.

You know how some little children have imaginary friends to keep them company and make them feel secure? Well, I'm not suggesting that you start introducing your positive voice to your friends and family as if she/he were standing there next to you. Rather, your healthy, positive voice will be there in your head to boost your morale and stand up for you when you just don't feel strong enough to stand up for yourself.

Walking the road to recovery becomes a lot easier when you have that positive voice walking with you, helping you to put one foot in front of the other.

There will be days when your negative voice is telling you you're not good enough, and you don't have the wherewithal to say, "Yes I am." But your healthy voice can come to your defense and say it for you.

Your healthy voice will always be there to have your back, to help you choose eating a meal over restricting, to lead you away from a triggering situation and to pick you up when you slip and fall and get you moving again. The farther along you get on the road to recovery, the stronger that voice will become.

Becoming Self-Considerate: Let Your Healthy Voice Take Care of You

One huge obstacle is that when you don't have enough love for yourself or your body, you tend to put yourself on the back burner and take care of everyone else first—that's how the backpack you've been carrying around got so heavy. You should not be number 101 in your list of 100 people you need to assist and support in this world. You need to put yourself at the top of that list. You deserve to be number one. Your healthy voice will help keep you front and center and make sure you take care of yourself—because if you don't, no one else is going to do it for you. True, there may be people to help you, but only if you put yourself forward and accept their help instead of shutting yourself off and shutting them out.

You should not be number 101 in your list of 100 people you need to assist and support in this world. You deserve to be number one.

Over my many years of therapy, I've been told time and time again that I needed to become a little more selfish and take time to take care of me. I always cringed when I heard the word *selfish* because it had so many negative connotations. I had a hard enough time feeling that I deserved anything at all, and now they wanted me to be selfish? Well, one of my mentors, Dr. Joann Hendelman, who is a brilliant psychologist specializing in the treatment of eating disorders, told me that instead of incorporating the word *selfish* into my recovery repertoire, I should start using the term *self-considerate*. Being self-considerate meant that it was okay for me to take care of myself and to take time just for me. It meant that I could consider my own needs while also considering the needs of others. In the recovery process you *must* be self-considerate, and your healthy voice will be the one to tell you that's okay. When your negative voice is telling you that you don't deserve it (or labeling it "selfish"), your healthy voice will be there to pipe up and say, "Excuse me, but she *does* deserve it and she *is* going to take care of herself." Then, down the road a bit, when you've been recovering for a while, your voice may be saying, "Hey, we're taking care of ourselves. We're being self-considerate."

The fact is that everyone deserves to feel good about him- or herself. At some point in the past we seem to have been told that we should always be striving for self-improvement, that there's always something we can change for the better—which is what helped many eating disorders, including my own, get started in the first place. And while it's certainly okay to try to do better, the issue for people with eating disorders is, once again, living with moderation. It's the lack of moderation—that black-and-white crayon mentality—that got us in trouble to begin with, and it's making friends with moderation and learning to use all the colors in the crayon box that's going to help us get better.

---

*Let your positive, healthy voice act
as your own personal cheerleader.*

It's good for everyone, not just people with eating disorders, to have a positive voice telling them, "You know what? You can do this, and you deserve it." Sometimes we're not able to do that for ourselves, and that's when we can let our positive, healthy voice act as our own personal cheerleader.

Pat Yourself on the Back

When I ask people if they've stopped to pat themselves on the back today, they tend to look at me as if I'd suddenly grown two heads. But the fact is, you need to do that. If you've taken a risk, if you've done the next right thing, you deserve a pat on the back. There won't always be someone there to praise you, so you need to praise yourself. This isn't being self-absorbed or egotistical—it is being self-considerate.

Again, it's not always easy. If you've ever tried to scratch an itch on your back and not quite been able to reach the right spot, you know how hard it can be. After years of listening to your negative voice, patting yourself on the back can sometimes be equally difficult. So this is something else your positive voice can do for you. Rosie, the Hulk, Elle, or whomever you've chosen as your ally in this struggle can be the one to give you that much-deserved pat on the back.

So, take a moment to evict that negative voice. Write up your classified ad and get it into the paper. There isn't any deadline, but the sooner you do it, the sooner you'll have a new, healthy internal friend. Nurture that voice and take it along with you so that it gets louder and louder, until it drowns out your negative voice. In the end, you will be left with a positive ally who contributes to and helps you through your journey of recovery and the rest of your life.

PROFILE IN RECOVERY:
Molly's Story

I remember the day Molly first called the office of the Alliance. As I spoke with her, I was immediately impressed by her insight and by the eloquence with which she spoke about her eating disorder. She told me that she had been recovering for the past seven years but that there were aspects of her eating disorder she had not been ready to give up entirely. Now, she said, the time had come. She was ready to be healthy, ready to be free, ready to be recovered. She began attending group and volunteering for the Alliance. Today I am honored and humbled to say she is an inspiration to me and to many other people in our group and throughout our community. I hope you will get as much inspiration from reading her story as I do from knowing her.

It is early morning when I open my eyes to see a blue blanket. There is a moment of confusion, and then I remember I am home. I am gripped by fear as I recall that I have left my life of independence and success in Brooklyn and am back in my family's home in Huntington, Long Island. I came home with the intention of staying one night to collect my thoughts, but somewhere inside I knew that would be much more complicated than anything I could imagine.

With this reality swimming through my thoughts, I glance around the tiny room that was once mine. *This is not my room anymore,* I tell myself over and over again. I am leaving very soon; everything is fine. I curl up under the covers and fondle my bones, convincing myself of these lies. I don't want to get out of bed, ever. Then I remember that my college roommate, Lily, is coming to visit me today. I have to bake an apple pie for her; it has to be ready before she arrives. I must move.

In the kitchen my feet are cold as I lay out my ingredients in perfect order: six red apples already peeled, butter, sugar, flour and a banana cake I made yesterday for a crumb topping. I have been baking incessantly for the past two weeks. Hours and hours of sleepless nights have been spent filling the house with food I refuse to eat.

....

Hours and hours of sleepless nights have been spent filling the house with food I refuse to eat.

....

While the crust cooks, I pace and squat, then run a sponge over the counter and table until the timer rings. I am standing over the pie, crumbling the banana cake topping, when my parents find me.

"What are you doing?" Mother asks.

"Baking a pie."

"For whom?" Her voice is tired.

"Oh, this is for Lily. She loves apple pie."

"Did she ask for a pie?" Mother asks.

"No." I reach for more banana cake to crumble.

"You need to stop baking now. Lily doesn't want an apple pie," Mother says.

"I'm surprising her. I'll stop after this one. I won't make anything else."

"No, Molly, it's time to stop *now*."

"No," I say, "I have to finish. Please let me finish." I start to cry.

"No, it's time to stop all this," Mother says again. I try to hold back the tears.

"Let her finish," Father says as he raises his hand, pivots and paces.

"It's time to stop baking. You don't have to finish," Mother insists. She is approaching me; she is going to touch me.

"Let me finish," I scream.

"No, Molly." She's holding my arms now.

"Why won't you let me finish?! I have to. Just let me," I sob as my body goes stiff.

"You don't have to," she says, her face close to mine.

"Yes, I do," I insist and arch away from her. "Stop touching me. No, no, no!"

"Yes, honey, it's time." Mother is rocking me now, rocking me out of my spell, and I can't stand it. "I love you," she whispers, and Father touches me.

"No," I explode. "No, you can't! Please don't...stop loving...let me just...no, I can't..." Nonsense words, over and over as I thrash, punching and biting, doing everything in my weak power to be free.

Lily did arrive that day, and my mother finished the pie. Lily thanked us for it, but that was not really what anyone cared about. My mother, father, my sister, Lily and I spent the entire afternoon sitting on the side porch. The sun was bright, but I was freezing, wrapped in a thick blanket. "Am I skinny, really skinny?" I asked again and again.

"Yes" was their answer. "You are very skinny and very sick." I knew that *sick* meant "crazy"; I knew that my life was changing forever. My secret was out.

That was the reality of my eating disorder ten years ago: prison, pain, no real comfort; just a slow, painful death sentence beyond the reach of anyone who dared to help. I was nineteen when my family intervened with meetings, self-harm plans, contracts, psychiatric hospitalization. My parents wrestled with me to comply, but I refused. My mom recently told me that when the scene I've just described transpired, she felt that I was no longer her child, that I had suddenly been possessed. What she did not know was that I'd been feeling that way for years, and she had just caught on. It was finally visible.

....

I knew that *sick* meant "crazy"; I knew that my life was changing forever. My secret was out.

....

During this time of family meetings and my indecision about whether or not I was willing or able to get well, I met Brian, my husband-to-be. Whenever he came to visit me, all I did was complain and ask him why he was bothering with someone like me. "Because I see a little light in you, I hear a little voice of reason," he would answer.

"There is no light. There is no voice," I would say.

After close to two years of feeling hopeless, waiting for someone or something to save me, I finally asked myself, *What the hell am I waiting for? Do I think this madness is just going to up and leave on its own?* I knew it wasn't that simple; I knew I would have to fight back, find that voice and scream. During those fragile days of a new beginning I asked Brian if he still heard that little voice of reason in me. He said I was listening to it, and I agreed.

I hit a plateau in recovery and remained there for about seven years, during which time I held on to this ritual or that rule, trying to negotiate a little eating disorder with a little health. I worked on my anxiety, depression, relationships, codependence and the other problems surrounding my eating disorder, until I finally came to believe that I deserved more than settling for a little health. I deserved to be free, and I knew that in order to free myself, I would have to give up the eating disorder. I would have to find that voice again, take off the muffler and let it sing so that others could hear it. There was a life out there that I was meant to live, and it did not involve an eating disorder.

Finally, three years ago, with so many healthy coping skills, so much to offer life, I felt like a flower kept under glass—desperate to bloom but feeling stunted. I wanted to be a mother and I knew that my eating disorder might deprive me of that chance. In desperation and with great hope I realized I didn't need to be restricted by the glass dome under which I'd been trying to survive. If I dared, I could break through that glass and grow free.

I believe I will always be growing. Some days will be wonderful, some just okay, and some days will be rotten—but I will be well, and that is living; that is what being in recovery means to me.

I called the Alliance for Eating Disorders Awareness, and Johanna assured me that I could recover. I threw away my scales, burned my calorie-counting books and did what my nutritionist asked me to do. I cried some days, and other days I laughed and rejoiced. I allowed myself to be human and be loved.

Some people say you will always be recovering. Well, I believe I will always be growing. I have a duty to be a good steward to my body and mind and to care for myself. Some days will be wonderful, some just okay, and some days will be rotten—but I will be well, and that is living; that is what being in recovery means to me.

The gifts of recovery are plentiful and keep coming. Just a few months back I was in a yoga class. There was a mirror and it was unexpectedly bright in the room. I followed my breath and prayed as I looked around the crowded class for a role model—someone who was strong, confident, peaceful and healthy, moving in concert with her spirit. And then my eyes met hers in the mirror. She was a sweaty, hot mess; she was beautiful beyond words; she was me. I had always been that woman; I just never knew it until I took off the blinders and looked inside.

··

> I looked around the crowded class for a role model—someone who was strong, confident, peaceful and healthy, moving in concert with her spirit. And then my eyes met hers in the mirror. She was a sweaty, hot mess; she was beautiful beyond words; she was me.

··

Today I have the privilege of helping others who are still imprisoned under glass and feeling unheard. I make eye contact; I see you; you can break through.

Thank you, Johanna, for believing in me and in recovery, for letting it be imperfect and fluid, for never capping the potential for growth. Thank you for giving recovery a voice and allowing me to scream its name: Towanda!

Chapter Nine

TALKING BACK TO IGNORANCE

A pessimist sees the difficulty in every opportunity;
an optimist sees the opportunity in every difficulty.
— SIR WINSTON CHURCHILL

THE WORLD IN WHICH WE LIVE is not recovery friendly. No matter how long you've been recovering or in recovery, you're going to run into people and situations that threaten to trigger your negative voice. I remember a time several years after I started the process when I had come to a point where I was ready to reincorporate exercise into my life. With the help of my recovery team, I had actually come to believe that it was possible to exercise in moderation— for health rather than weight loss—and that if I did decide to work out, I didn't have to work out compulsively.

I was still a bit apprehensive, because exercise had been so much a part of my eating disorder for some time, but I gathered up all my tools and went to a local gym to sign up for a membership. As part of the incentive for joining the gym, I became the lucky recipient of two sessions with a personal trainer who, I was told, would familiarize me with all the gym equipment and determine what kind of program suited me best. I scheduled the appointment and met the trainer who would be assisting me. He was a big, buff guy with huge pecs and triceps, and the first words he said to me were, "So, what are you here for?" And without giving me a moment to answer, he continued, "Are you here to lose a few LBs?" At first, I promise you, I had absolutely no idea what he was talking about, and I must have looked confused, because he went on, "We're going to lose some pounds, right? We're going to trim you up." And, of course, the first thing that popped into my mind was my negative voice telling me, "Oh, he's telling me I'm fat." But I immediately called up my healthy, positive voice and told him, "No, I am not here to lose weight. I'm here to incorporate a healthy exercise regimen into my life." (Yes, I had practiced that little speech several times with my therapist just in case a scenario like this should arise.) So I told the trainer that my goal was to take care of myself and be healthy. To which he replied, "Well, you know, a possible side effect is that you *do* lose weight." So I reiterated as forcefully as I could, "That's truly not what I'm here for. I'm really here for my health."

Objectively, I could understand why the trainer was saying those things. I'm sure that many, if not most, of the people who join a gym do so to make good on a New Year's resolution to lose weight, and he was undoubtedly telling me what he thought I wanted and expected to hear. But he wasn't listening to me. So then he said, "Okay, let's just put you on the scale and see where we are." At that point I was really starting to lose my patience. I was using my voice, being loud and clear, and this guy was still not hearing me. I was very grateful to be far enough along in my recovery at that point not to let this guy trip me up and send me right down to the bottom drawer. But the whole situation was honestly starting to make the hairs on the back of my neck stand up. I told him I really didn't need to know what I weighed, and he said, "Why? You *should* know your weight. We can use that as a starting-off point and to monitor your progress." Once again, much louder this time, I stressed that I was doing this for *health!* "*I am doing this for my health! My health!*" That was when he got out the fat calipers. No, I am not joking. This man obviously didn't have a clue—and didn't *want* to be clued in—about who *I* was or what *I* wanted. He had no ability to change his focus and truly hear what I was saying.

Finally, I just explained as clearly as I could that while I understood why he was so insistent on weighing me or using his funny little machine to measure my body fat, I was recovering from an eating disorder. I was really there for health and wellness. I was taking care of myself, and knowing my weight and how much body fat I had was not going to help my recovery. I was not going to let a number on the scale have power over me anymore. At that point he nodded knowingly and said, "Well, that's all good, but don't you want to know what you weigh?" Needless to say, I threw my hands in the air, left the gym, wrote a letter to the corporate office and never returned.

People Aren't Mean; They're Just Ignorant

About four years ago, a woman in our group shared an experience she'd had several days before our meeting: she had been at a doctor's appointment and explained her history with bulimia to her new physician. When she finished, he'd looked at her and said, "You know, you should get over this pretty quickly. It's not a big deal. All you have to do is start eating and not throw up." Amazed at his response, not to mention his ignorance and arrogance, she said that all she had wanted to do in that moment was punch him in the face. But she knew that violence wasn't actually an option, so she tried to explain her struggle as forcefully as she could. "The only word I could think of to account for his behavior was *ignorant*," she said. "I just wished that I had an Ignorant stamp so that I could stamp it on his forehead. That way, every time I looked at him, I'd see the word *ignorant* in front of me, and his words would hold less weight in my mind. What he said wouldn't be such a trigger for me."

We all laughed and commiserated with her, and that's how the concept of the "Ignorant stamp" was born. We all need to remember to carry an imaginary Ignorant stamp, the kind you use with an ink pad, in our purse or our pocket, because at some point we are going to encounter people who are plain ignorant and just don't get it. I often hear people say that those who have never had an eating disorder cannot know what the struggle is like, and that's true. You can talk and explain until you're blue in the face what it's like to battle an eating disorder, and there are still going to be people out there who believe you *chose* to have an eating disorder and, therefore, you can now *choose* to start eating again and "just get over it." Much like that doctor, they often believe it's not a big deal.

We all need to remember to carry an imaginary Ignorant stamp in our purse or our pocket, because at some point we are going to encounter people who are plain ignorant and just don't get it.

One comment I hear quite regularly that always has me pulling out my Ignorant stamp faster than I can blink is "Oh, I wish I could have an eating disorder for a month or two." What? Are you kidding me? It never ceases to amaze me that our society really does glorify and glamorize what I fought for so long to get rid of. Another equally ignorant comment is "Oh, wow, you're so skinny. You're so lucky!" Clearly, these people have no idea how much some of us are struggling.

That's their problem, but it becomes your problem when you allow these ignorant people to trigger negative thoughts and unhealthy behaviors. You need to make sure that they do not have power over your recovery. If you remember to get out your trusty Ignorant stamp and aim it right at the middle of their forehead, it will be a lot easier for you to say (not out loud, of course), "You just don't understand. You're ignorant. I'm not giving you any space in my head. You don't pay rent. You don't deserve to have any power over me at all, and I think it's time for you to move out!"

We Live in a World Full of Ignorant Messages

According to Dr. Jean Kilbourne, an internationally recognized authority on alcohol and tobacco advertising, as well as the image of women in advertising, the advertising industry is a more than 200-billion-dollar-a-year business. On average, individuals are exposed to more than three thousand advertising messages a day, which means that we each spend about three years of our life watching, reading or hearing ads. And what are the majority of the advertisements for? You got it! Cosmetics, skin firming creams, gels, tanning products— that is, products to enhance our appearance. Or diet and weight-loss programs and products. Or food!

The diet industry alone is a 40-billion-dollar-a-year industry, so you can be certain that those who are selling these products are doing just about everything in their power to get their message out. Doesn't it seem that everywhere you turn a celebrity or a sports star is trying to sell you an "easy, get thin quick" secret? They're hard to avoid.

In truth, those of us who are in recovery from an eating disorder, trying to take care of ourselves, do the next right thing and be healthy, are living in an environment that's extremely hostile to recovery. All around us, people are constantly telling us they can make us prettier and thinner—the underlying message is clear: we'll never be thin enough or pretty enough without their help. And that's just reinforcing what our negative, eating disorder voice has been telling us all along.

Those of us who are in recovery from an eating disorder, trying to take care of ourselves, do the next right thing and be healthy, are living in an environment that's extremely hostile to recovery.

To combat those messages, you need to rely on your healthy voice, along with all the other tools you've gathered so far. And now you can add the Ignorant stamp to the arsenal of tools in your recovery chest. Make sure you have it with you at all times so that you can pull it out (metaphorically, of course) whenever you need it.

I actually had real Ignorant stamps made to give out to the people in my groups as holiday gifts. I put them in little velvet bags and told our group members to carry the stamp with them so that it would be available whenever they were confronted by an ignorant and potentially harmful comment. I have to admit that over the years, when I have encountered particularly triggering people or situations, I find myself reaching into my purse and feeling for the stamp as a reminder not to be taken in or taken down by them. I continue to give Ignorant stamps to the members of my groups, and I had to smile when one woman said she would just keep on using her imaginary stamp. She didn't want a real stamp because, she admitted, she didn't trust herself not to stamp people who were truly ignorant with real ink.

Sometimes They're Just Worried or Trying to Help

Have you ever sat at the table with "caring" friends or family members who just stared at you and, every time you picked up your fork, let out a sigh or a gasp or sucked in their breath in anticipation? I know they're just worried, but are those sound effects really necessary? I don't think so! It is hard enough to take healthy steps without an audience giving you a not-so-subtle play-by-play commentary.

———————————

It was hard enough for me not to think about my eating disorder constantly, and having those around me obsess over it as well was giving me no respite whatsoever. I wanted them to acknowledge the other parts of my life that made up my true identity, not the false identity of the eating disorder.

———————————

For a long time while I was recovering, my mother called every day to ask what I'd eaten for lunch. I know she was concerned about me because, let's face it, she had come very close to losing her child, and it made her feel better to keep on asking. But at that point I was trying to *not* make food the focus of my life, and finally one day I just had to say, "You know, Mom, I love you and I really appreciate your concern, but I need you to trust me now. I need you to trust that I'm going to take care of myself. Maybe you could call and just ask me how my day is going instead of asking me what I ate." I needed my mother to shift her focus from my eating disorder to other aspects of my life. It was hard enough for me not to think about it constantly, and having those around me obsess over it as well was giving me no respite whatsoever. I wanted them to acknowledge the other parts of my life that made up my true identity, not the false identity of the eating disorder.

I know that trust takes time (I had to learn to trust my own body, which I'd always been so uncomfortable with), and I know it was particularly hard for my mother, knowing how much I'd manipulated her and lied to her in the past, to learn to trust me again. But I needed that trust from my mother, as well as from the others who cared about me, and gradually I've earned it.

Listen with Your Healthy Ears

A few years ago, during the holiday season, a group of volunteers and I were running a gift-wrapping booth at a local mall to raise funds for the Alliance. I was feeling very grateful to the members of my support group who had given their time to help raise awareness and money for the organization. As we went about our task, many people would come up to the counter, read the sign stating that "All Proceeds Go to Benefit the Alliance for Eating Disorders Awareness" and share stories about how eating disorders had affected their lives. They talked about family and friends who had recovered, those who were still struggling or those whom they, sadly, had lost to the disorder. But there were also those who had no idea how serious eating disorders really are. I distinctly remember a woman who came up to the counter to have an item wrapped, looked at our sign, then looked from me to a support group member who was also wrapping, and said, "Well, it's obvious neither of you has a weight problem." Then she stared straight at my fellow volunteer, who was still on her journey to recovery, and said, "You are so lucky to be so thin." I knew how potentially triggering that comment could be for someone who was trying her hardest to take care of herself and be healthy, so I immediately reached into my purse and handed her my Ignorant stamp. She looked at me, smiled and said, "Don't worry. I'm good. I already visualized myself stamping her forehead with my imaginary stamp."

In truth, almost *anything* anyone can say about weight is capable of triggering negative thoughts when you're recovering from an eating disorder. If someone says, "Oh, it's great to see you looking so healthy," your eating disorder ears might hear, "Wow, do you look fat." If someone says, "Oh, it's so great to see that you've got your appetite back," you might hear in your head, "Uh-oh, she's telling me I ate too much."

> *In truth, almost* **anything** *anyone can say about weight is capable of triggering negative thoughts when you're recovering from an eating disorder.*

In fact, one of the women in our support group recently fell into just that trap. She said that when she'd run into a neighbor whom she hadn't seen for a while, he'd remarked, "I'm happy to see you looking so great. You look like you're at a healthier weight." She told the group that when she heard that, she'd "flipped out." At that point another member of the group chimed in, saying, "Wait a minute, isn't that your goal? Isn't that why we're here?"

And, of course, that supportive group member was right. The rational part of our brain may know that we're supposed to be striving for a healthy weight, but the negative, irrational part is saying, "Oh my gosh, I'm fat!" We know that food is the best medicine and the first order of treatment for an eating disorder, even though we may not want to process that thought. What the woman in my group needed to do was take a step back and ask herself, *What do you think you would have preferred him to say? "Gee, your self-esteem is really looking vibrant"?*

Sometimes, when our negative voice is in control, we're just looking for more negatives to fuel the fire. There may be many good things happening or said to us, but we're tuning them out. All we're picking up on are the things that validate our own negativity. What we need to do is become more conscious of seeking out the positive and dismissing the negative so that the next time someone compliments us on looking healthier, we can simply say, "Thank you. That's my goal," and give ourselves a pat on the back.

Our negative ears have a sneaky way of distorting the things we hear, so that when someone tells you one thing, you may hear something entirely different— like a bad version of the game of Telephone. We need to make sure that what we are hearing is actually what's being said. One tip that has been very helpful to me is when I'm talking with someone I really trust and with whom I feel safe, I ask him or her, "Do you mind if I just repeat back what you've said to be sure I understood you correctly?" Now, whenever I feel that someone has said something triggering, I start my response with "So what I am hearing you say is…," and I repeat what I heard (or thought I heard). Very often, when I do that, the other person will stare at me in amazement, wondering, *How did she get that from what I said?* So the next time someone tells you how healthy you look, check out what your negative ears might be hearing by saying, "So, what I am hearing you say is that I look fat." Checking out what you just heard validates your healthy voice and helps to quiet your negative voice.

Maybe you've been in a restaurant when someone in the booth behind you or at the next table says to one of his or her eating companions, "You know, you really shouldn't be eating all that fattening food," or "Do you know how many calories that has?" Whether it's about the diet du jour, good food versus bad food or the diet someone is going to start "tomorrow," diet and weight-loss talk has become central to most social situations. But for people who are trying to recover from an eating disorder, even though the person wasn't talking to them and the remark had nothing to do with them, it can be a trigger. Their negative voice twists what was overheard and turns it into fuel for a negative flame. The trick is to smother the flame before it has a chance to flare up by using your tools, including your Ignorant stamp.

And the trigger doesn't always have to be spoken. One woman in our support group told us about the time she arrived at work to discover that her office mates, many of whom were dieting, had placed a scale in the kitchen, directly in front of the refrigerator. They thought that seeing the scale would make them think twice about eating, but for her this was like her biggest nightmare come to life. She didn't know what to do, and I suggested that she had four options:

1. Avoid the problem entirely by never entering the kitchen again.
2. Go in the kitchen, feel extremely anxious and potentially give power to your negative voice.
3. Break into the office in the middle of the night, steal the scale and throw it in a Dumpster.
4. Politely let your office mates know that having the scale in front of the refrigerator is making you feel uncomfortable, and ask them to move it (or even suggest that they discard it altogether).

Clearly, option four would be the most positive (please do not break into your place of employment). I also explained to her that there was no need to get into specifics about why the scale made her uncomfortable. We don't all know everything about other people's lives, nor do we need to.

And sometimes the negative remark might actually be directed at you, even by someone you know loves and supports you. In that case it's perfectly okay for you to say, "You know, I understand and appreciate your concern, but what you said isn't really helpful to me." You need to speak up and use your voice. It's perfectly acceptable—even essential—to establish and maintain healthy boundaries and to be self-considerate.

But sometimes you may not be far enough along in your recovery to use your voice. Instead you may just play the remark over and over again in your head like an endless negative tape. If a negative remark has taken up residence as an unwelcome roommate in your head, you need to evict it. You need to press the Stop button and eject the tape. Sit down and write the person a letter explaining why you are mad, hurt, annoyed or whatever you are feeling. Instead of holding on to those feelings, get them out on the paper. No one is going to read this, so please do not get caught up in writing the "perfect" letter. Just let your thoughts and feelings flow. When you are finished, take your letter into the kitchen, put it in the sink and light a match to it. As you watch it burn, let the ignorant words you heard go up in smoke.

You need to speak up and use your voice.
It's perfectly acceptable—even essential—
to establish and maintain healthy boundaries
and to be self-considerate.

Every time you can take the opportunity to educate even one person about the reality of eating disorders, you're doing something to eradicate the ignorance that's out there—one person at a time. Sometimes you will be effective, and other times you will encounter people who are simply not able to listen and truly hear you. When that happens, you can always get out your Ignorant stamp.

The most important thing, however, is *always to listen with your healthy ears and carry your Ignorant stamp with you at all times.* As the famous American Express slogan states, "Don't leave home without it."

Chapter Ten

BRIDEZILLA MEETS BRIDEOREXIA AND OTHER TRIGGERING OCCASIONS

Where there is love there is life.

—MOHANDAS K. GANDHI

ONE OF THE BEST THINGS I EVER did for myself, other than choosing recovery, was to get back on a horse—literally. Several years before that happened, I had taken my younger cousins horseback riding. They loved it, but unfortunately, when we accelerated from a casual walk to a gallop, I was thrown, and from that moment on I vowed never to get back on a horse. Well, as I would soon come to find out, never say never!

A few years later my then boyfriend, Max, said that we needed more outdoor fun in our lives and that he would like us to go horseback riding. My immediate reaction was to say, "Great. Have a good time. Enjoy the scenery. Call me when you get back." But he kept insisting and assuring me that we'd have a great time. Trust me, I tried every excuse in the book, but to no avail. Max was adamant, telling me that it was going to be great and well worth my time. Finally, on the appointed day, I woke up with butterflies in my stomach and left the house for the stable. I was terrified, but everyone was being incredibly nice to me, so I climbed up on my assigned horse and we took off at a slow walk. There were six in our little group, with the ride leader directly in front of me and Max right behind. After a few nervous minutes, I actually started to really enjoy the trail ride.

Before I could say yes, all that was going through my mind was how grateful I was for having chosen recovery and for having lived to experience this moment, for having been given a second chance at life.

After a while, the trail leader turned to me and asked what I did for a living. When I told her about the Alliance, she shook her head and let me know that several young riders at her stable were currently struggling with eating disorders. As we were nearing the end of the trail, she asked if we could ride a few minutes longer without the rest of the group so that we could continue our conversation. I asked if it would be okay for Max to join us, and she said, "Of course. I'm sure he'll enjoy it. Besides, I want to show you both the prettiest part of the trail." When we arrived at that spot, the leader told us we absolutely needed to take a picture and capture this moment, so Max dismounted and walked up to me (while I was still on my horse). He pulled out an engagement ring, told me I was the love of his life and asked me to spend the rest of my life with him. He'd planned the whole thing in advance with the woman from the stable, but I was taken totally by surprise. In fact, I was, quite literally, speechless (I know, me speechless—doesn't happen often). Before I could say yes, all that was going through my mind was how grateful I was for having chosen recovery and for having lived to experience this moment, for having been given a second chance at life and for all the people who had supported me on my journey—and, above all, for having met this man who had taken the time to know me, eating disorder and all, and who was now my greatest supporter, my friend and my biggest fan.

Eight years before, when I was still entrenched in my eating disorder, I could never have imagined this day ever happening for me. Having so little self-love, I could never have imagined that anyone would love me. In fact, I wasn't even sure that I'd still be around eight years later. So I was sitting on that horse, staring at the ring in Max's outstretched hand, and all this was going through my mind until finally he said, "Um, hello? Are you going to give me an answer?" You already know what my answer was. He helped me dismount, and I threw my arms around him and said yes about a dozen times. Back at the stable, we got off our horses and went home to start making phone calls to our friends and family.

The Madness Begins

It was only a few hours later that my whole world seemed to turn upside down. From "Congratulations. I'm so happy for you," the responses I was getting to my big announcement turned to "What are you going to wear?" "How are you going to do your hair?" and "Are you going to get a spray tan?" It seemed that all anyone wanted to know was how I planned to be or do this or that. It was no longer about our impending marriage but about an event— the wedding itself. And then, no more than a week later, people started to tell me *they* needed to lose weight or buy a dress or change their hairstyle for *my* wedding.

No more than a week later, people started to tell me they needed to lose weight or buy a dress or change their hairstyle for my wedding.

I'm sure that most little girls have, at some point, imagined what their wedding day would be like. We imagine the flowers we'll be carrying, the gown we'll be wearing, the song that will be played for the first dance and maybe, just maybe, we even imagine what the groom will look like. I have to admit, I'd done that, too. And I certainly had plenty of ideas about how I thought I should look and what I would wear as a bride. But mainly, at that point, I was pretty comfortable in my own skin and simply thrilled that I now got to reap this reward for all the hard work I had done. Getting married was one of the long-term goals I had set for myself all those years before, one that I had been able to reach because I was healthy.

Going for the Gown

A few months into the engagement, I was in Manhattan with my aunt and cousin when my aunt said, "Since we're here in New York, why don't we go shopping for a wedding dress?" I can't say that I wasn't a bit apprehensive, because, after all, this was the day when you're supposed to look the best you've ever looked in your life. But I was also looking forward to seeing myself in all those gowns. After being the eternal bridesmaid, it was my turn to go shopping for a bridal gown, and I was excited. So we made an appointment at a very chic bridal salon, and off we went.

It was Easter week, and there had been one of those freak spring snow-storms in New York, so I was wearing jeans, a peacoat and my Converse sneakers. When we entered the salon, the first thing the lady at the reception desk said to me was, *"You're the one getting married?"* I guess most brides-to-be dress up more for their big shop, and I suppose I could have taken the remark to mean "You look much too young to be getting married," but I didn't. I took it as a criticism, and it rattled me a bit, but I brushed it off as best I could and dutifully followed my assigned saleslady (who was much more elegantly dressed than I) into a dressing room. She asked me several standard questions, such as my wedding date, the type of wedding I was planning and what I envisioned my dress would look like. Then she told me to get undressed and said she would bring in the gowns for me to try on.

The saleslady looked at me and said,
"Honey, you are going to lose weight
before the wedding, aren't you?"

Again, I was a bit anxious, but I told myself that people who are healthy and happy in their bodies have no problem getting undressed in front of total strangers (hmmm). So I stripped down to my undies and a moment later the saleslady reappeared—carrying a piece of shapewear. She wanted me to wear body armor under my wedding gown! I tell you, everywhere I turn, that indestructible body armor seems to reappear. (Luckily there was no fireplace around this time.)

The first gown she brought in was one I had seen in a magazine. It was absolutely beautiful, and although I knew it was well beyond my price range, I wanted to try it on anyway. I took a deep breath and stepped into it, and that was when the worst of all my fears came true. The saleslady looked at me and said, "Honey, you *are* going to lose weight before the wedding, aren't you?" My aunt, sitting in the corner of the spacious dressing room, yelled out, "Oh, my goodness," while my cousin just sat with her mouth open, looking like a frightened deer caught in the headlights. I wish I could tell you that my healthy voice spoke up immediately and defended me, but she didn't. Suddenly my negative voice was taking up every inch of space in my head, and my healthy voice was nowhere to be found. I was so overwhelmed that I just wanted to run away and hide. But I didn't.

Suddenly my negative voice was taking up every inch of space in my head, and my healthy voice was nowhere to be found. I was so overwhelmed that I just wanted to run away and hide.

After telling me that the dress was not great on me, the saleswoman brought in another gown, and this time she remarked that my body was too "boxy" for the dress. "Thank you so much for sharing that!" I wanted to scream but didn't. With the third gown she started to make comments about my arms. It was at that point, as I was standing in the dressing room, wearing my borrowed body armor, with the gown half on and half off, that I looked directly at her, called upon every tool in my recovery arsenal and said, "I have to stop you right there. I'm in recovery from an eating disorder, and had I not been as far along in the process as I am, what you just said could have been extremely destructive for me. I've been waiting for this moment for twenty-eight years, and you have now successfully ruined it. Next time you want to offer your input on other people's body types, I suggest that you stop and think before you say anything, because you never know what that person is going through or has been through. I came here to buy a dress, but unfortunately, I will not be needing your services, after all. Thank you for your time." Mentally, I not only slapped her with an Ignorant stamp but imagined a flashing neon arrow pointing down at her and illuminating the word IGNORANT. Then I got dressed and left. As I was walking out, I passed another bride talking with her bridal consultant about how much weight she had lost since her engagement day.

I called upon every tool in my recovery arsenal and said, "I'm in recovery from an eating disorder." Mentally, I not only slapped her with an Ignorant stamp but imagined a flashing neon arrow pointing down at her and illuminating the word IGNORANT.

Truth to tell, I didn't go wedding-dress shopping again for another four months. Luckily for me, it was a long engagement.

Messages from the Bridal Industry and Others

Like most prospective brides, I went online and registered for a few bridal Web sites. That was when the unsolicited tips and advice about how to lose weight and what's the best way to look good for your wedding really started to flood not only my e-mail inbox but my mailbox as well.

I began to think about all the other brides who were in my situation, women who had struggled and recovered not only from eating disorders but from disordered eating and a distorted body image, and who now wanted to stay healthy throughout the wedding planning process. I started to surf the bridal message boards to see what was really going on out there. The first thing that struck me was how disordered even relatively healthy people suddenly become around their wedding day. Among other things, I discovered that, on average, women buy their wedding gown two sizes too small and use it as a motivator to reach their desired weight-loss goal. Years later, I had to laugh when I watched the 2009 film *Bride Wars*, in which one character says to another, "You don't alter [designer] Vera [Wang] to fit you. You alter yourself to fit Vera." All I could think was, *How fitting!*

No matter where I looked, what I read or whom I spoke with, the conversation was never about the actual marriage; it was all about how I was supposed to look on my wedding day. There was more advice than you could shake a stick at about everything from tanning options to bridal Botox to every quick-weight-loss diet that's ever been invented. I even received a coupon from a plastic surgeon offering a complimentary bridal liposuction treatment if I purchased a full-price tummy tuck. *What?* Every day, I was being bombarded by "fun" e-mails suggesting I try this bridal boot camp or that "bridal drink" that would help me lose X number of pounds before my "big day." Several Web sites sent out daily e-mails intended to inspire and support future brides on their journey to achieving their dream body transformation. Some sites even awarded members gold stars to act as reinforcers based on how much weight they had lost. And one photographer knowingly informed me that, after all, I'd have these pictures for the rest of my life. (Yes, and hopefully there would be many more pictures after that, I silently reminded myself.) Needless to say, I had to buy extra ink for my Ignorant stamp.

I have to admit that all this diet talk started to get to me. If so many people were going on diets for my wedding day and I thought they already looked great, maybe I should be dieting, too.

But it wasn't just the wedding industry doing this; it was also all the people around me—family and friends—who announced they were going on diets. And it wasn't even their wedding. I have to admit that all this diet talk started to get to me. If so many people were going on diets for my wedding day and I thought they already looked great, maybe I should be dieting, too. I had to work overtime to make sure my healthy voice was at every wedding meeting and family get-together, and more than once I left the dining table in order to remove myself from a potentially triggering conversation.

Bridezilla or Brideorexia?

I think it is safe to say that we've all become familiar with the term *Bridezilla* (a difficult, unpleasant, perfectionist bride who creates unnecessary aggravation for her family, friends, bridal vendors and even her groom). But you may not be so familiar with another new bridal term, *Brideorexia*. Yes, it's a real word and an all-too-real phenomenon. It was coined to describe women who lose weight at a dangerous rate or in unhealthy ways in advance of their wedding. Not only is this type of behavior not frowned upon, but it is often directly and indirectly encouraged by the 86-million-dollar-a-year bridal industry.

According to a 2008 study by Lori A. Neighbors and Jeffery Sobal published in the journal *Appetite*, more than 70 percent of brides want to lose weight before their wedding day, and more than one-third of them use such extreme measures as prescribed medications they obtain illegally, diet pills or supplements, going on liquid or other extreme diets, fasting, taking laxatives, or skipping meals to achieve their idealized wedding-day weight. One Web site (Bride.net) tells the story of a woman who almost died from drastically limiting her caloric intake as she was preparing for her wedding and consulting a pro-anorexia Web site for information about how to diet most effectively.

One member of our own support group had been pretty comfortable with her body and didn't develop an eating disorder until she became engaged.

One member of our own support group had been pretty comfortable with her body and didn't develop an eating disorder until she became engaged. Then she started to look through bridal magazines, was getting the same e-mail messages I had received and began to think that maybe she *should* lose some weight before her wedding. She'd ordered her dress, and when she took it to be fitted, the seamstress, who was an older European lady, patted her on the stomach and said, "I'm glad to see that you're not one of those girls who loses so much weight for her wedding. It's good to see you looking so full and beautiful." That was all she needed to decide that she *absolutely* had to lose weight. She went on a diet, the pounds started to come off and before she knew it, she wanted to lose more and more. It never felt like she had lost enough. Because, again, eating disorders aren't about the weight. The weight loss just numbs and covers up the emotions or feelings that are too difficult to deal with. That seamstress's innocent comment was the trigger that set off her eating disorder.

Stay Focused and Just Say No

It isn't easy—believe me, I know. Those months leading up to my wedding probably put more obstacles in my path than anything else I'd encountered since my recovery. But I'm happy to say that I never went off course. There were times when I had to reach out and ask for guidance, but thankfully, my support system came through and I never lost my way.

Despite all those months of being urged to focus on how I would look when my "special moment" finally arrived, when I was actually walking down the aisle, I wasn't thinking about what I looked like, how my dress fit, how much I weighed or even about that little pimple on the base of my chin. Instead, I took the opportunity to really soak up the moment. Amazingly, what I *didn't* see were people criticizing my appearance, as I had done so many times in the past. What I saw (with my healthy eyes) were my parents beaming with love, the faces of the many loved ones who had walked next to me on my journey to recovery, my amazing friends (the epitome of floaties) and, most of all, the amazing man who was waiting for me under the chuppah and gazing at me with love.

*The greatest thing about recovery is that
there is a whole life, filled with infinite
possibilities, after your eating disorder.*

After the wedding there's a whole life still ahead of you, and the greatest thing about recovery is that there is a whole life, filled with infinite possibilities, after your eating disorder. Recovery rocks! In fact, it's better than anything I could ever have imagined.

Whatever the Occasion, Keep Your Eye on the Prize

While many of us think of our wedding day as one of the biggest occasions in our lives, there are many other "big events"—whether it be a new career, a new school or moving to a new location—that could threaten to sidetrack you. Those are the times when you *must* put on the equivalent of horse blinders so that you keep your eye on the prize—your health and only your health—instead of being distracted by everything that's going on in your peripheral vision. The minute you allow your mind to wander, you're unlocking the door and giving your negative voice just that tiny opening it needs to sneak in and take over.

I don't know about you, but getting through Thanksgiving, which we all know is the year's biggest pig-out holiday, was difficult for me when I first started recovering from my eating disorder. In fact, it's almost become a rule that you're supposed to eat as much as you can on Thanksgiving and then crawl to the couch moaning that you're totally stuffed, can't eat another bite and are never going to pig out again. And then your aunt Joyce comes in with the warm apple pie, so, of course, you find room and have a slice of that, too — with ice cream, of course.

The first Thanksgiving after starting my recovery process, I was at my parents' house. I'd gone to my therapist and talked about what I'd be comfortable with eating and what risks I would take. We talked about boundaries and how I would handle this potentially triggering situation. The family was seated around the table, and I knew I was making good choices about what I was eating. I was feeling pretty good about myself, and, having listened to my hunger, I decided to ask my mother for a bit more of the mashed potatoes. Well, you would have thought I'd just won the lottery or invented the cure for some mysterious disease. Within seconds, fourteen pairs of eyes were focused on me, and everyone at the table started to exclaim in two languages, "Oh my goodness, voilà! Johanna asked for seconds! *C'est magnifique!* How wonderful!" Everyone at the table threw their hands up in the air, rejoicing, and I…well, I pretty much flipped out. The last thing I wanted to do at that moment was to eat the food now sitting on my plate. I left the table immediately and stayed in my room for the next few hours. I know my family's reaction came from a place of love, but why did they need, once again, to bring so much attention to the food and my eating behaviors? Couldn't they have just smiled inwardly? To keep myself from becoming overwhelmed, I mentally pulled out my Ignorant stamp and used it liberally, if only in my mind.

But Thanksgiving isn't the only time families can inadvertently trigger negative feelings. There's Christmas, Chanukah, birthdays, or the Fourth of July picnic — whenever families tend to come together, there's always the possibility that your aunt Fanny or uncle Joe will say something that is potentially triggering. It happens to everyone; you don't have to have an eating disorder to be triggered by a foolish or thoughtless remark.

When that happens, you need to pull out every one of your tools to support yourself as you continue to do the next right thing—and don't be afraid to use that Ignorant stamp when you need it. This is one day, one night, one moment in your life, and you have the rest of your life to live and be healthy.

Afterword

RE(DEFINE) (REAL)ITY™

*Sometimes it's the smallest decisions that can
pretty much change your life forever.*

—FELICITY PORTER, "PILOT," *FELICITY*

THE REALITY IS THIS: there is a life beyond your eating disorder. What you get from recovery is your life back, but it's not the life you set out to create; it's different from anything you could ever have imagined and much, much better. It's not perfect, it's got its ups and downs, but it's real and it's wonderful.

The reality is this: there is a life beyond your eating disorder.

If you had asked me at the age of twenty or twenty-one where I saw my life in ten or twelve years, I would have had to say that, honestly, I saw no life. My eating disorder *was* my life. It was my everything: my best friend and my worst enemy, my floatie and my sinkie. I couldn't imagine a life without my eating disorder, much less a life in which I would be thriving.

None of us chose to have an eating disorder,
but we all get to choose to recover.
We get to decide that we deserve *to recover.*
We get to choose to live.

My journey has been a roller-coaster ride, but one of the most important discoveries I've made is that no one ever needs to be ashamed or embarrassed about having an eating disorder. None of us choses to have an eating disorder, but we all get to choose to recover. We get to decide that we *deserve* to recover. We get to choose to *live*.

I Define What's Real

Eight years ago, I was in the dining room of my parents' house with my then seven-year-old cousin, who was standing with her hands on the table, sucking in her stomach. When I asked her what on earth she was doing, she told me that she wanted to look like a very famous singer whose image appeared on the cover of every popular magazine at that time.

As I was recovering, and now that I'm recovered, it made me very sad that we live in a world where little boys and girls aspire to look like the extremely airbrushed and sometimes very unhealthy celebrities they see every day in the media. We are constantly bombarded with unrealistic images of what we're supposed to look like, and then when we fall short—which we will, because they *are* unrealistic—we feel bad and punish ourselves for being unable to achieve the impossible. All our lives we've been told that it's okay to hate ourselves, it's okay to be dissatisfied with the bodies we have, and that we should always be striving for better. What we need to learn instead is that it's okay to feel *good* about ourselves and be grateful for the bodies we were given. It's okay to value our health and be satisfied with our choices.

We are constantly bombarded with unrealistic images of what we're supposed to look like, and then when we fall short, we feel bad and punish ourselves for being unable to achieve the impossible.

What I ask people in my groups, and am now asking you, is to please take a step back from those unrealistic ideals and start being real. To achieve that end I have created a movement called re(Define) (Real)ity, which encourages people to imagine a world where loving themselves for who they are and as they are can become a reality.

That said, however, what's real for me may not be the same as what's real for you, so I ask you to take a good look at yourself and try to believe that you absolutely do deserve much better than whatever your eating disorder has been telling you. Look at your strengths, be proud of who you are and give yourself that pat on the back you deserve.

*All our lives we've been told that it's okay
to hate ourselves, it's okay to be dissatisfied
with the bodies we have, and that we should
always be striving for better.*

Recovery Means Steering Your Own Course

When you're in thrall to your eating disorder, you're really just a passenger on your own life's journey. The car of life is on cruise control and you simply go where it takes you. Recovery means climbing over the central console, taking back control of the wheel and steering your own course. In the process, you may take a few wrong turns because you're in foreign territory, but the wonderful truth is that we each have our own built-in GPS, and eventually it will get us back on the right road. It may take a few recalculations to determine what that road is, but in the end, you will find your own true north.

Me 101

Going through the whole recovery process is like taking a course in Me 101, turning the microscope on yourself and discovering what you really want. That sounds scary, I know, but it's also extremely rewarding. The more clearly you are able to see your long-term goals, the better you will be able to appreciate the fact that recovery *is* worth it.

Do you remember the woman in one of my support groups who changed the personification of her healthy voice from her grandmother to her unborn child? When she began her journey, she couldn't imagine ever being healthy enough to bear a child. Over the next two years she came to group faithfully and worked with a wonderful nutritionist and a great therapist. Her journey had peaks and valleys, but over time I could see that she was getting stronger and stronger, and taking the steps she needed to take care of herself. Finally, one day she said that she was beginning to believe recovery was worth it, and that she was happy she'd been willing to take the risks she needed to take in order to be healthy. This, of course, made me cry. When another group member asked her what had happened to change her mind, her whole face lit up as she said, "I'm pregnant." In effect, she had achieved her long-term goal and come to realize that whatever it had taken to get there, it was worth fighting for. And, I am happy to report, during the time I was writing this book, she gave birth to Rowan, a beautiful, healthy baby girl. What a gift!

Take a step back from those unrealistic ideals and start being real.

As I've said, my own goal from the very beginning has been to help others along their path to recovery and to bring more attention to the terrible toll eating disorders are taking on so many individuals every day. When I founded the Alliance and began using my voice for the first time, something shifted inside me. The more presentations I gave, the more tenacious, willing, terrific women I met in my support groups, the stronger I became. Now, whenever I hear someone say, "I can't do this," my positive, healthy voice proclaims, "Oh, yes, you can!" that much louder. And you really can. You can reclaim your life. You deserve this.

The work I've done through the Alliance has given me more validation and reinforcement than anything I could have imagined. I truly see it as the best gift I have ever been given in my life. On my own journey through my eating disorder and throughout my recovery, I have been blessed to meet the most amazingly strong, courageous and devoted people. When I stopped dancing all those years ago, I never thought that I would ever find anything that filled my heart the way ballet did. But I was wrong. The work I do today is my passion—it's my reward and it's my mission.

Now, whenever I hear someone say,
"I can't do this," my positive, healthy voice
proclaims, "Oh, yes, you can!" that much
louder. You can reclaim your life.

The first time I went to Washington with a delegation from the Eating Disorders Coalition in 2003, I found myself sitting in an office across from a member of Congress and realized that I, too, had a voice, and I deserved to be heard (as do all those millions of people who are battling eating disorders in silence every day). That is a powerful feeling, but no more fulfilling than being able to walk alongside another person on the road to recovery, as I am privileged to do with the members of my groups every day.

Accept the Gift That Is Offered

My grandmother once told me this popular story based on Loren Eiseley's *The Star Thrower*: A little boy is walking on the beach with his father. The beach is littered with starfish and as they walk, the boy picks up one starfish after another and throws it back into the ocean. After a while, his father asks what he's doing and the little boy says, "Throwing the starfish into the water. The sun is up and the tide is going out. If I don't throw them in, they'll die." "But," says his father, "don't you realize there are miles and miles of beach and there are starfish all along every mile? You can't possibly make a difference." "But," the boy replies as he bends down and throws another starfish into the ocean, "I made a difference to that one."

There is *someone—even if you aren't aware of it right now—who will be so honored to walk next to you on your journey. All I am asking is that you be willing to ask for help.*

Getting your life back is the most precious gift I can imagine. And there are people out there who, like that little boy, want to give you that gift. Sometimes, when you're struggling, it's hard to believe that. It's hard to believe you deserve the help they are willing to give you. And sometimes it's hard to see where to turn. But you do have directional signals inside you; you just need to pay attention to them. Pick up the phone, call a national eating disorders organization and ask for a referral. Consult the Getting Help section in the back of this book. Take someone with you to your first appointment if that's what you need. There *is* someone—even if you aren't aware of it right now—who will be so honored to walk next to you on your journey. All I am asking is that you be willing to ask for help.

What I Wish for You

At the end of every one of our support groups, I ask each person to name something for which he or she is grateful, and then I ask everyone to turn to the person next to them and make a wish for that person. I have to admit that this is my favorite part of group. So, as we conclude our time together, I would like to say what I am grateful for and make you a wish for your journey back to you.

I am grateful for the opportunity to recover, for all my amazing, devoted floaties who never let me sink, for having the willingness to take the next step, for the ability to get up when I tripped and fell, for all the diversity of colors in my crayon box of life, for being able to both give and fully receive love, for trusting my support team enough to let them be my eyes and ears when I couldn't trust my own and, most of all, for the opportunity to be a fellow traveler on other people's journeys of recovery.

---

*My wish for each of you is that you come
to believe you truly do deserve to get better,
that you deserve to be happy and healthy
and that you will take not only the first step
on your own journey to recovery but
also the second, third and fourth,
and every step you need to keep on going.*

My wish for each of you is that you come to believe you truly do deserve to get better, that you deserve to be happy and healthy and that you will take not only the first step on your own journey to recovery but also the second, third and fourth, and every step you need to keep on going. I wish that you will use all the tools in this book and discover others of your own. I wish that you will make that phone call and reach out for help when you need it. And most of all, I wish that you come to believe you *are* worth it, that you are fabulous just the way you are.

PS: As you come up with new tools and add them to your personal toolbox, I invite you to go to our Web site, www.eatingdisorderinfo.org, click on the Contact Us button at the bottom of the home page and share your new tools so that we can share them with others. None of us can ever have too many tools in our box.

Getting Help

FINDING THE THERAPIST WHO'S RIGHT FOR YOU

MANY PEOPLE HAVE ASKED ME what they should ask when speaking with a potential psychologist/therapist/nutritionist/etc., and my advice is, first of all, have a list of questions and don't be afraid to ask them. Some of the questions I believe to be essential are:

- How much experience have you had working with eating disorders?
- What percentage of your practice is devoted to people with eating disorders?
- What kind of professional training do you have? Education? Licenses?
- What do you charge for a session? Do you have any kind of sliding scale?
- Do you take insurance? Which plans?
- What is your therapeutic approach?
- Do you work with a treatment team?
- What are your goals for treatment?

Many people want to know how long the treatment will last, but no therapist can really tell you that because, as you should know if you've read this book, the road to recovery is different for each individual.

And, finally, you need to know that even the greatest therapist in the world may not be a great therapist for you, just as no one outfit is the perfect fit for everyone. If you feel that the first—or second or even third—person you see doesn't feel like the right fit, don't be afraid to make a change. If it isn't working, you have no obligation to stay. And don't think that just because the first person you saw didn't work out, no therapy is going to work. You should also keep in mind, however, that therapy isn't a tea party, and being uncomfortable is going to be a part of getting better. So before you make a decision to change therapists, ask yourself honestly where that feeling of discomfort is coming from.

There are many, many wonderful practitioners out there who are ready, willing and able to become one of your floaties and help guide and direct you through the journey of recovery.

If you don't know where to start, please pick up the phone and call one of the following amazing organizations for a referral in your area.

Resources

AED: Academy for Eating Disorders

111 Deer Lake Road, Suite 100
Deerfield, IL 60015
www.aedweb.org
Phone: (847) 498-4274
E-mail: info@aedweb.org

For eating disorders professionals. AED promotes effective treatment, develops prevention initiatives, stimulates research and sponsors an international conference.

ANAD: National Association of Anorexia Nervosa & Associated Disorders

www.anad.org

Help Line: (630) 577-1330

General: (630) 577-1333

ANAD was officially launched in 1976. It is the oldest eating disorder organization in the nation. ANAD distributes listings of therapists, hospitals and informative materials and sponsors support groups, conferences, advocacy campaigns, research and a crisis hotline.

Andrea's Voice Foundation

www.andreasvoice.org

Andrea's Voice is dedicated to promoting education and understanding aimed toward the prevention, identification, diagnosis and treatment of disordered eating and related issues.

Anna Westin Foundation

PO Box 268

Chaska, MN 55318

www.annawestinfoundation.org

Phone: (952) 361-3051

E-mail: kitty@annawestinfoundation.org

The Anna Westin Foundation is dedicated to the prevention and treatment of eating disorders. The Foundation is committed to preventing the tragic loss of life to anorexia nervosa and bulimia and to raising public awareness of these dangerous illnesses.

BEDA: Binge Eating Disorder Association

550M Ritchie Hwy, #271
Severna Park, MD 21146
www.bedaonline.com
Phone: (410) 570-9577
E-mail: info@bedaonline.com

BEDA is an international organization that includes individuals with the disorder, family and friends, and multidisciplinary practitioners. BEDA's mission is to raise awareness, educate and provide resources for its members and the general public.

A Chance to Heal

PO Box 2342
Jenkintown, PA 19046
www.achancetoheal.org
Phone: (215) 885-2420
E-mail: info@achancetoheal.org

A Chance to Heal prevents the incidence and reduces the impact of eating disorders and promotes the importance of a positive body image by educating and influencing parents, young people, educators and health-care professionals.

Dahlia Partnership

PO Box 50071
St. Louis, MO 63105
www.dahliapartnership.org
Phone: (314) 726-1503

The Dahlia Partnership is a collaborative organization of professionals and volunteers dedicated to improving the early diagnosis and treatment of people with eating disorders, increasing access to care and strengthening family and community support.

EDA: Eating Disorders Anonymous
www.eatingdisordersanonymous.org

Eating Disorders Anonymous is a fellowship of individuals who share their experiences, strength and hope in order to solve their common problems and help others to recover from their eating disorders. Meetings are held throughout the United States and internationally.

EDANJ: Eating Disorders Association of New Jersey
10 Station Place
Metuchen, NJ 08840
www.edanj.org
Phone: (800) 522-2230
E-mail: info@edanj.org

The Eating Disorders Association of New Jersey is a statewide nonprofit organization whose mission is to provide supportive services and resources, such as support groups, referrals, speaking engagements, advocacy and more, to individuals affected by eating disorders, including family members and friends.

EDC: Eating Disorders Coalition for Research, Policy and Action
720 7th Street NW, Suite 300
Washington, DC 20001
www.eatingdisorderscoalition.org
Phone: (202) 543-9570
E-mail: manager@eatingdisorderscoalition.org

The mission of the Eating Disorders Coalition for Research, Policy and Action is to advance the federal recognition of eating disorders as a public health priority. Its goals include raising awareness among policy makers and the public at large about the serious health risk posed by eating disorders; promoting federal support for improved access to care; increasing resources for research, education, prevention and improved training; increasing funding and support for scientific research on the causes, prevention and treatment of eating disorders; promoting initiatives that support the healthy development of children; and mobilizing concerned citizens to advocate on behalf of people with eating disorders, their families and professionals working with these populations.

EDCT: Eating Disorders Coalition of Tennessee

2120 Crestmoor Road, Suite 3000
Nashville, TN 37215
www.edct.net
Phone: (615) 831-9838
E-mail: contactus@edct.net

The Eating Disorders Coalition of Tennessee brings together professionals and community members dedicated to educating, empowering and supporting those affected by disordered eating.

Eating Disorder Foundation

3003 East Third Avenue, Suite 110
Denver, CO 80206
www.eatingdisorderfoundation.org
Phone: (303) 322-3373

The mission of the Foundation is to be an effective resource for both the general public and the health-care community in the collective effort to prevent and eliminate eating disorders. The Foundation engages in education and advocacy initiatives together with timely support and help in identifying appropriate treatment options for individuals with eating disorders and their families.

EDIN: Eating Disorders Information Network
600 Means Street, Suite 100
Atlanta, GA 30318
www.myedin.org
Phone: (404) 816-3346
E-mail: info@myedin.org

The Eating Disorders Information Network is a nonprofit organization dedicated to the prevention of eating disorders, including anorexia, bulimia, compulsive overeating and other forms of disordered eating, through education, outreach and action.

EDN: Eating Disorder Network of Maryland
25 W. Chesapeake Avenue, Suite 202
Towson, MD 21204
www.ednmaryland.org
Phone: (410) 339-3474
E-mail: ednmaryland@gmail.com

The Eating Disorder Network of Maryland is a community organization aimed at helping individuals, families and professionals learn more about eating disorders. The organization offers support groups, community outreach, professional education and an online referral database.

Elisa Project
3102 Oak Lawn Avenue, Suite 520
Dallas, TX 75219
www.theelisaproject.org
Phone: (866) 837-1999
E-mail: tep@theelisaproject.org

The Elisa Project educates individuals, families and the medical community about eating disorders and the importance of a positive body image.

F.E.A.S.T.: Families Empowered and Supporting Treatment of Eating Disorders
PO Box 331
Warrenton, VA 20188
www.feast-ed.org
Phone: (540) 227-8518
E-mail: info@FEAST-ED.org

Families Empowered and Supporting Treatment of Eating Disorders is an organization of and for parents and caregivers to help loved ones recover from eating disorders by providing information and mutual support, promoting evidence-based treatment and advocating for research and education to reduce the suffering associated with eating disorders.

F.R.E.E.D.: Gail R. Schoenbach Foundation for Recovery and Elimination of Eating Disorders
18 Chestnut Hill
Warren, NJ 07059
www.freedfoundation.org
E-mail: gail@freedfoundation.org or kathleen@freedfoundation.org

The Gail R. Schoenbach F.R.E.E.D. Foundation is a nonprofit organization dedicated to eradicating eating disorders. Funds contributed to the foundation provide individuals with the financial support needed for the treatment of eating disorders.

H.O.P.E.: Helping Other People Eat
7850 St. Andrews Circle
Orlando, FL 32835
www.hopetolive.com
Phone: (321) 231-0791
E-mail: allisonkreiger@yahoo.com

Helping Other People Eat strives to educate all age groups about the warning signs, symptoms and side effects of eating disorders and offers informa-

tion, tutorials, references and public speakers to aid in eliminating eating disorders.

IAEDP: International Association of Eating Disorders Professionals

PO Box 1295
Pekin, IL 61555-1295
www.iaedp.com
Phone: (800) 800-8126
E-mail: iaedpmembers@earthlink.net

A membership organization for professionals that provides certification, education, local chapters, a newsletter and an annual symposium.

Kirsten Haglund Foundation

PO Box 2592
Farmington Hills, MI 48333
www.kirstenhaglund.org
E-mail: misskhaglund@gmail.com

The mission of the Kirsten Haglund Foundation is to provide hope, networking and financial aid to those seeking treatment and freedom from eating disorders.

MSF: Manna Scholarship Fund

1325 Satellite Boulevard, Suite 703
Suwanee, GA 30024
www.mannafund.org
Phone: (770) 495-9775, Ext. 107
E-mail: info@mannafund.org

Manna Scholarship Fund is a nonprofit organization dedicated to providing funds for residential and inpatient eating disorder treatment for individuals lacking insurance coverage or for those with inadequate insurance coverage. MSF grants scholarships to recipients by providing direct payment to partnering eating disorder treatment facilities.

MEDA: Multi-Service Eating Disorders Association Inc.

92 Pearl Street
Newton, MA 02458
www.medainc.org
Phone: (617) 558-1881
E-mail: info@medainc.org

MEDA is a nonprofit organization whose mission is to prevent the continuing spread of eating disorders through educational awareness and early detection. MEDA serves as a support network and resource for clients, loved ones, clinicians, educators and the general public.

NEDA: National Eating Disorders Association

601 Stewart Street, Suite 803
Seattle, WA 98101
www.nationaleatingdisorders.org
Phone: (206) 382-3587
Hotline: (800) 931-2237

NEDA is the largest not-for-profit organization in the United States working to prevent eating disorders and provide treatment referrals to those suffering from anorexia, bulimia and binge eating disorder and those concerned with body image and weight issues.

Ophelia's Place

PO Box 621
Liverpool, NY 13088
www.opheliasplace.org
Phone: (315) 451-5544
E-mail: hope@opheliasplace.org

Ophelia's Place is a nonprofit organization committed to empowering individuals, families and communities to redefine beauty and health through initia-

tives that increase self-esteem, improve body image and introduce alternatives to dangerous desires for perfection by providing outreach, advocacy and educational services to those impacted by eating disorders, disordered eating and body dissatisfaction.

Index

thinness as desired, 39
unrealistic images, 184–85

D

Dahlia Partnership, 196

Diary of a Young Girl, The (Frank), 41

diversifying your recovery funds, 115–16

dresser drawers. See "How Many Drawers Are in Your Dresser?"

E

Eating Disorder Network of Maryland (EDN), 199

eating disorders
control issues and, 12, 13, 14, 17, 18, 20, 21, 23, 27–28, 36, 37, 42, 46, 49, 62, 64, 65, 76, 103, 110, 128
black-and-white thinking, 25, 26, 44, 49–50, 70, 73, 91, 92–93, 111, 112, 125, 146
danger of trading one addiction for another, 111–12, 116, 120
emotional component, 25, 46, 57, 179
environmental or lifestyle choices and, 38–39, 118
as fake security blanket, 110, 126
fear of giving up, 22, 25, 30, 57
genetic component, 36–40, 76, 92, 118
identity and, 22, 83, 89–90, 91, 99, 117, 119, 184
ignorance about, 157–59
lack of people in treatment for, 2
mortality rate of anorexia, 2
negative voice of, 3–4
number of people with, in the U.S., 2
perfectionism and, 9, 13, 23–24, 32, 42, 47, 52–53, 92, 120, 129
power of, 3
as safe haven, 65, 81, 117, 124
triggers, 27, 31, 32, 96, 169–82

Eating Disorders Anonymous (EDA), 197

Eating Disorders Association of New Jersey (EDANJ), 197

Eating Disorders Coalition for Research, Policy and Action, 2, 33, 188, 197–98
Eating Disorders Coalition of Tennessee (EDCT), 198

Eating Disorders Foundation, 198

Eating Disorders Information Network (EDIN), 199

Eiseley, Loren, 188–89

Elisa Project, 199

emotions
facing fears, 72
fears and recovery, 89–90, 128
feeling bad as familiar, 134
Feeling Words or Feeling Faces exercise, 131–35
gradual immersion in, for recovery, 55–58
suppression or numbing and eating disorders, 14, 20, 23, 24, 25, 46, 49, 57, 128–29, 179
underlying eating disorders, 25, 46
"What Would You Do If You Weren't Afraid?", 51

exercises. *See* recovery exercises

F

fake security blankets, 103–22
danger of trading one addiction for another, 111–12
distinguishing between positive blankets and, 109–10
eating disorder as, 110

Families Empowered and Supporting Treatment of Eating Disorders (F.E.A.S.T.), 200

Feeling Words or Feeling Faces exercise, 131–35

Felicity, 183

Frank, Anne, 41

Fried Green Tomatoes (Flagg), 137, 142

G

Gail R. Schoenbach Foundation for Recovery and Elimination of Eating Disorders (F.R.E.E.D.), 200

Gandhi, Mohandas K., 169

genetics, 36–40, 76, 92, 118
family members with eating disorders, 39–40

goals of recovery, 48

Gold, Tracey, 17

guilt, 14, 36, 38, 40

Acknowledgments

My mother always taught me that, in life, when a door closes, you should always look for a window. This book is perhaps one of my biggest windows of all, and I know that without the love, support, guidance and encouragement of many people, this would not be a reality.

To my parents, Jacqueline and Bernard Kandel: You have given me life time and time again. There aren't enough words to tell you how much I love you and how grateful I am to call you my parents. Thank you, Dad, for always pushing me to be the person you always knew I could be and, Mom, for being the kindest, most warmhearted person on this earth. You are my heroes.

To my grandmother Rosalie Belilty, who is one month shy of her hundredth birthday: Thank you for always teaching me that there is nothing I cannot do. Thank you for being my healthy voice and proving to me that there are angels on earth.

To Sarah Pelz, editor (and friend) extraordinaire: Thank you for believing in me and this project from before day one. I know how lucky I am to have worked with someone as phenomenal as you. Thank you for your vision and hard work. You are simply fabulous!

To Judy Kerns: Thank you for walking next to me on this journey and for representing me (and my voice) so beautifully. I am forever grateful to you and your talent.

To the amazing team at Harlequin: Thank you for honoring me with a More Than Words Award in 2008 and for letting me speak in Toronto. I remain humbled. You are all so talented, and I am extremely fortunate to work with such a great company.

To Adrienne Ressler: Thank you for writing such a beautiful foreword. It is a privilege for me to work with you and to know you. Thank you for all your contributions to the field of eating disorders and body image.

To Allison, "Jasmine," Jamie and Molly: Thank you for contributing your incredible stories of recovery to this book. I am so honored to call some of the most inspiring people in the world my close friends. You are true warriors.

To the best "floaties" in the world, my family and friends! I love you forever!

To my family: Bella, Edith, Gerard, "Bug" (Alison), Julian, Valerie, Cedric, aka Spider-Man (Pigeons Rule), Thierry, Sebastien *et tout ma famille en France et Israel* (all my family in France and Israel)—*Je vous aime!*

To Richard, Esther, Sosha, Zev, Vivian and Lionel Zaretsky: Thank you for welcoming me with open arms into your family. I consider myself so very lucky. I love you!

To Barbara and Karla, my family, although not through blood but through lots of love, history and friendship.

To my Biche, aka Jennifer B. (love you always and forever), Jesse Blah (our shining star), Garrett Swann (PS I love you), Autumn (co-prez, Black Cloud Association), SMS (Dr. Sarah), Rachelle (secret friends), Jillian, Kim B (CSI— like the TV show), Lee Ann (I heart LITM), Jill Terral, Coley K, my boys Michael (Denise) Shauger and Dana Campagna, Raquel, Sara and Henry Harary, Suzanne, Sara, Ashley, Summer, Melissa and Jennifer (NSYNC 4ever), Sandy C (I miss you) and *all* the phenomenal people I am lucky enough to call my friends. You have taught me the meaning of true friendship through-out the years.

I have been blessed with two of the best mentors in the world: Dr. Marie Shafe, thank you for helping to direct me back to health and ultimately back to me and, Dr. Joann Hendelman, thank you for being so dedicated to the Alliance, this book and mostly to our friendship. Your constant support and feedback are a true blessing.

Thank you for your love. Big hugs!

To my goddaughter, Isabella: May you grow up to love and respect yourself the way that we love you today and always.

To *all* the members of my treatment team throughout the years: I thank you for leading the way and being my eyes when I wasn't yet able to see the path in front of me.

To the board of directors, teen advisory board and volunteers of the Alliance: We would not be in existence without you!

To Mrs. Joan Eigen, for believing in me and the Alliance from day one: Your support enabled our organization to become and remain a reality.

To Suzette Wexner and Palm Healthcare Foundation, for welcoming me with open arms into your "family" and being so supportive of me and the Alliance.

To my heroes Kathleen MacDonald, Jeanine Cogan, Kitty Weston and the Eating Disorders Coalition: Thank you for giving me a platform to use my voice to help make a difference.

To all the people who are currently on the journey to recovery: Never give up. Help is available and recovery is possible. You deserve to be healthy and happy.

To all the amazing women who have attended Monday Night Support Group throughout the years: You are so brave and inspire me every day. This book is dedicated to you.

And last, to my husband, Max Zaretsky: I am the person I am today because of you. You are my gift. Thank you for never running away, for never giving up on me, for always supporting me and mostly for loving me to the moon and back (and back). *Je t'adore.*

About the Alliance for Eating Disorders Awareness

In October 2000 the Alliance for Eating Disorders Awareness (the Alliance) was created as a source of community outreach, education, awareness and prevention of the various eating disorders currently plaguing our nation. Our aim is to share the message that recovery from these disorders is possible and that individuals should not have to suffer or recover alone. We seek to educate individuals about the dangers of this epidemic and to reduce the rate and severity of eating disorders for people of all ages.

The Alliance offers various programs and services throughout the state of Florida and nationwide and advocates for change in eating disorders legislation. Since its inception, the Alliance has made presentations on eating disorders and their prevention to over 110,000 individuals. We strive to promote a healthy body image, aid and empower those currently struggling and instill a sense of self-love, self-acceptance and self-confidence. Through presentations, seminars, workshops, phone and e-mail support, treatment referrals, support groups and informational packets, we offer opportunities for individuals to receive the information they need free of charge.

Mission Statement

The Alliance for Eating Disorders Awareness (the Alliance) is a nonprofit organization working to prevent eating disorders and promote a positive body image, free from weight preoccupation and size prejudice. We accomplish this through educational presentations, cutting-edge information and referral, training, advocacy, support and mentoring services.

re(Define) (Real)ity

A movement to:

1. celebrate diversity
2. challenge artificial ideals
3. empower yourself
4. define *real*

Can you imagine a world where loving yourself can be a reality? We can; re(Define) (Real)ity is a movement created by the Alliance that challenges society to embrace diversity, dismiss unrealistic ideals and prove that beauty comes in all shapes and sizes. It's time to get *real!* To join the movement, please visit www.redefinereality.org.

Community Education

The Alliance is committed to increasing education and awareness through educational presentations at public and private middle schools, high schools and colleges, and for graduate programs, social service agencies, youth groups, health-care programs, etc. We will also individualize a specific program to meet your needs. Evaluations of programs are available upon request.

Professional Training

Individualized professional training in the areas of diagnosis, treatment, advocacy, working with various age groups, co-occurring disorders and the like is available through the Alliance to educators, mental health practitioners, all health-care providers and other community groups and agencies. Evaluations of programs are available upon request.

Support Groups

Our support groups are designed to provide an environment in which those who are suffering from and those whose lives are affected by eating disorders can express their feelings and experiences to trained individuals who understand their personal struggles. The Alliance provides a free weekly support group for females ages eighteen and over, as well as a monthly Friends and Family Support Group.

Advocacy

The Alliance is committed to the improvement of education, outreach, treatment and research pertaining to eating disorders. Through regular trips to state capitals and Washington, DC, letter-writing campaigns, phone calls/e-mails and training of other advocates, we work to be a voice for change. The Alliance is a proud member of the Eating Disorders Coalition (EDC) and the National Eating Disorders Association (NEDA) STAR (States for the Treatment, Access, and Research) Program.

Referrals

The Alliance is committed to providing the community with referrals to local eating disorders specialists (physicians, therapists, nutritionists, etc.). As such, we are constantly working to update our referral network with the most recent information about local, specialized practitioners.

About the Author

JOHANNA S. KANDEL, WHO RECOVERED after a ten-year-long battle with various eating disorders, is the founder and executive director of the Alliance for Eating Disorders Awareness, based in West Palm Beach, Florida. Since its inception in 2000, the Alliance has brought information and awareness about eating disorders to more than 110,000 middle school, high school and college students nationally. In addition, Johanna runs free weekly support groups, mentors women with eating disorders through their treatment and recovery, helps thousands of people to gain information and find the help they need, and advocates for legislation on the local, state and national levels.

She is a member of the Eating Disorders Coalition Junior Board, Florida co-team leader for the National Eating Disorders Association's STAR Program and a member of both the Board of Directors and Expert Advisory Committee for Girl Future, a Web site dedicated to educating and empowering girls ages nine to fifteen. She is an active participant in National Eating Disorders Awareness Week, has received many awards for her ongoing support and advocacy work, including the Jefferson Award for Public Service and Harlequin Enterprises' More Than Words, and has appeared on national television programs, including NBC *Nightly News* and *Today*.

She lives in West Palm Beach, Florida, with her husband, Max Zaretsky, and her dog and cat, Sammie and Leela.